fertile
THINKING

ANYA SIZER WITH CAT DEAN

fertile
THINKING

*Your practical and emotional aid
through the trials of infertility ...
and beyond*

First published in 2010 by
Infinite Ideas Limited
36 St Giles
Oxford
OX1 3LD
United Kingdom
www.infideas.com

A CIP catalogue record for this book is available from the British Library

ISBN 978-1-906821-55-5

Cover designed by Cylinder
Text designed and typeset by Nicki Averill
Printed and bound in Great Britain by Bell & Bain Ltd, Glasgow

CONTENTS

ACKNOWLEDGEMENTS

Our grateful thanks go to Andrew Sercombe for championing the book from the start and allowing us to use his Powerchange exercises, to Mia Aimaro Ogden for her excellent editing, and to Julia Bueno, The London Women's Clinic, More to Life and INUK for their support and enthusiasm.

From Cat: To my friends and family, thank you for believing me when I said it would happen. Mike, I couldn't have done it without you. Thank you. And to Thomas – for being my little inspiration.

From Anya: Thank you to everyone who helped us through, especially Romey, who always told me there would be a family out there – we would just have to fight for it. This book is dedicated to my two miracles, Hope and Barney, who beat the odds to get here and were worth every part of the battle. To God, for getting me through. And to my husband and best friend who means the world to me. I love being a family with you.

INTRODUCTION

My name is Anya Sizer and I am the proud mum of two IVF children – children we were given odds of 1 in 125,000 of ever conceiving. Six long years of infertility treatments, thousands of pills, hundreds of needles and five rounds of IVF later, we know that statistics don't always tell the whole story.

My journey began in January 2001 when, very excitedly, I came off the pill and looked forward to a few months of trying to conceive before the inevitable blue line appeared on the pregnancy test.

Eight months later, I had begun to get impatient and just a tiny bit apprehensive, so I managed to get our doctor to agree to some initial tests. A precaution, I thought, to reassure us that everything was okay. How wrong I was.

My initial blood-test results were normal, but there was a problem with my husband Damion's sample – no sperm at all were detected – a condition called azoospermia. We were given the news by a doctor who, without looking up from his notes, simply said: 'Mr Sizer, you are completely infertile and it is highly unlikely you will ever have children.'

That evening, Damion went to bed and pulled the duvet over his head, refusing to talk, while I launched into an Internet fact-finding mission exploring every possibility. Both of us felt isolated, sad and incredibly scared that the doctor's words would be the end of the story. However, we soon entered the weird and wonderful world of assisted reproductive technology (ART).

From December of that year to May of the next, we both went through test after test; my hormone levels, womb lining and fallopian tubes were examined, and Damion underwent an exploratory operation to see why he wasn't producing any sperm. We also endeavoured to get ourselves into the best shape possible and followed a very specific healthy-eating plan, as well as both seeing counsellors and getting all the support available to us.

In June, we saw one of the UK's top gynaecologists to get advice on our next steps. He was kind but to the point. IVF (in vitro fertilisation) wouldn't work in our situation and our odds of conceiving through ART were approximately 1 in 125,000. In his opinion, our options were donor sperm or adoption only. The days that followed were bleak and, as a couple, we felt almost at breaking point. Why was this happening? Would we ever get through it?

We took a few weeks to reassess, and came to the unpopular (with others, that is) decision that 1 in 125,000 just might be worth a go. After all, what if we were that 1? So, in July 2002, we started our first IVF cycle.

It is hard to explain just how exhausting and overwhelming the whole process of IVF can be, and how much strength you need to keep going, both physically and emotionally.

During this first cycle, the doctors discovered that, in addition to Damion's issues, I turned out to be what they describe as a 'poor responder'. Put simply, my body didn't respond well to the drugs and I produced only four eggs – a small yield for someone in my age bracket. But again, we were determined that one egg and one sperm were all that was needed.

On the day of egg collection, Damion also had to have an operation, to see if any sperm could be found in his testes, a possibility even with azoospermia.

We almost expected to go home with bad news, but the impossible happened – not only were sperm found, but they were immediately injected into the four eggs that had been harvested from me. So somewhere downstairs in the hospital, in a small Petri dish, were four sets of potential life. Lying there, recovering from general anaesthetic, we were both absolutely stunned. We were in the race.

Then we began the two-week wait. I always found this time the hardest part of an IVF cycle. Finally, though, I bought a pregnancy test, and it really felt like life would never be the same, whatever the result. But two strong lines quickly appeared. I was pregnant. It had worked.

In April 2003, our daughter was born. There was only one name that really fitted: Hope. She was our first miracle, at odds of 1 in 125,000.

Eighteen months later, we began to think about extending our family and, for the next eighteen months, experienced one loss after another: one IVF miscarriage, two failed IVF cycles and, strangest of all, an unsuccessful natural pregnancy.

That time was hard and we felt increasingly desperate and isolated; some of our friends and family, understandably, began to wish we could just settle for the miracle we already had.

In December 2005, we decided to do our last IVF cycle before exploring adoption. This cycle was by far the most intense as not only had they diagnosed my poor response as an indicator of early menopause, but they had also detected a potential immune issue. With the azoospermia, too, this meant our odds were even worse than when we had begun.

Once again, I responded poorly to treatment, and twice during the cycle I was advised to consider giving up entirely. I felt this was the end of the line, but nonetheless I continued with the embryo transfer. This time, during the two-week wait, I felt nothing, and as I went into the clinic for the blood test, I told Damion I would call him later on to confirm it was a no.

To everyone's amazement, not least mine, the pregnancy test was a very strong positive reading and, as I walked in to collect the results, the staff all cheered, knowing just how huge a battle we had won.

In August 2006, our second miracle was born: a baby we called Barnaby, meaning 'son of comfort'.

Our road to parenthood was certainly one of the most difficult things I have ever been through and, to this day, I still feel incredibly privileged and blessed to be a mother. I now work with couples who are going through IVF, using coaching to support, encourage and equip them for every stage of their journey. I see clients individually, and run workshops and a fertility support group. My goal in this book is to provide you with some of the tools I give to my clients to help them live full and positive lives while they're going through treatment. In writing the book I enlisted the help of my long-time friend, Cat Dean, who is a journalist, writer and Powerchange coach. She helped me to transfer my thoughts onto the page and also helped to choose the exercises.

One of my favourite quotes from the Bible is, 'Comfort others with the comfort you have received'. I feel so privileged to be able to live that today and I hope you receive comfort from your reading.

CHAPTER 1

EQUIP YOURSELF: ESSENTIAL COACHING TOOLS

"The future depends on what we do in the present."
Mahatma Gandhi

Why are you here? I don't mean in a philosophical way, although that's also an interesting question; I mean, what made you decide to pick up this book? What do you expect to find? What would be most helpful for you right now? Clients who come to me for coaching have a variety of motivations and expectations about the process, but usually have one thing in common – a burning desire to have a child. They may be at the beginning of their journey and want to maximise their chances of becoming pregnant, or they may have reached the end of their tether after several years of failed fertility treatments.

A quick search on Amazon brings up more than 46,000 matches for 'fertility' books – there's a lot of information, as well as money to be made, in the baby-making business. I remember when I first started out on my quest for motherhood and things weren't going quite as quickly as planned. I scanned the shelves of my local bookshop, hoping for something to provide the answers I was so desperately seeking. There is a lot of advice and information out there, and it can sometimes feel overwhelming. But there was little that met my emotional needs, or that encouraged me to see the bigger picture beyond my diet, hormones and sex life. I'm not saying that it's not crucial to arm yourself with as much knowledge as possible to increase your chances of getting pregnant, but I needed something that would help me look beyond my 'problems' and encourage me to see myself as more than just a reproductive system. That is what I promise to do for you.

My approach

One of the first things I tell my clients is that I'm not medically trained, although I have extensive experience of the IVF process. While cognitive behavioural therapy (CBT), coaching and other mind/body programmes have been proven to increase your chances of success, my ultimate aim as a coach is for you to feel like a whole person by the end of the process. I can't promise you a pregnancy – it would be totally unethical of me to offer such an impossible guarantee – but I can help you gain a feeling of control over your life and a renewed sense of self, both of which are so easily lost during the challenging journey of fertility treatment.

It is also worth remembering that I am a coach, not a counsellor. While coaching has now become an established and respected profession, many people are still confused about the difference between coaching and counselling. Put simply, counselling usually focuses on the past and the reasons why you are feeling the way you do today. Coaching focuses on how you are in the present and the changes you need to make in order to achieve the future you want. While, inevitably, there is some overlap, as clients often find that the process of coming to terms with their fertility issues can bring up uncomfortable emotions from the past, my aim is to bring the focus to the present and to ways you can help yourself regain control of your life.

If a client appears to be clinically depressed or cannot manage their strong emotions sufficiently to deal with their present behaviour, I will always refer them to a specialist counsellor or psychotherapist.

You may also want to go and see your GP who can refer you for treatment on the NHS. I believe that counselling is important and definitely has a place when you are going through fertility treatment. Likewise, as you go through the exercises in this book, you may experience unexpected feelings and encounter issues from your past that you had not anticipated. If these feel overwhelming for you and you need additional support, you may choose to seek the help of a professionally trained psychotherapist or counsellor (see Further Resources at the back of this book).

What you will need

This book is designed to be a supportive resource for you as you undergo your journey and there is no requirement for you to spend money on additional gadgets and gizmos. I believe there are already too many people out there desperate to capitalise on women's desire to have children. At the back of this book I list resources that I and other people have found helpful. Some are free; there is a charge attached to others. But I do not believe that you need to spend a fortune in order to give yourself the best chance of living a full life. All you will need to complete this book is a notebook and a pen, and a willingness to look at yourself and your situation in a whole new way.

Where you are right now?

Jot down the answers to the following questions in your notebook. You don't need to spend too long thinking about them, just write down whatever comes to mind.

- What has brought you to this book today?
- What have the past few months been like for you?
- What would you like to get out of this book?

■ Are you looking for a practical approach or a more emotional one?
■ How do you see yourself right now?

At this stage, we are looking to establish a picture of where you are today, without judgement, blame or criticism. It is so easy to spend our lives in the past (*if only, why didn't I?*) or the future (*what if?*), but in order to put ourselves in a strong position to live a full life in the present, we need to know what we're up against.

How did it feel to answer those questions? Is there anything else you need to add to complete the picture of how you are today?

Exercise: the best-friend technique

Often when we're going through a difficult time, we struggle to see the full picture, as we're trapped by our thoughts and feelings. One technique that can help pull you out of the trap is to imagine that a close friend or family member is in your situation. What would you say to them right now – what advice, support and reassurance would you give them? Write it down.

Dealing with feelings

Keeping a journal

My clients often find writing to be a useful tool in helping them to deal with their emotions. And the great thing about keeping a journal is that you don't have to be a Booker Prize-winning writer to benefit because nobody but you will be reading it. It doesn't even need to make sense for it to work. Research into the power of keeping a journal in improving health is conclusive. An American study[1] of patients with asthma and rheumatoid arthritis found that nearly half experienced a 'clinically relevant' improvement in symptoms after four months of writing about stressful experiences. The researchers concluded that the brain deals with traumatic memories in a different way from everyday thoughts, and that the anxiety caused by these can result in 'physical and biological dysfunction'. Getting it all down on paper helped the patients to process the memories and change the way they felt about the trauma, which, in turn, had a profound physical effect on their health.

Buy yourself a notebook to use exclusively for the purpose of writing down your feelings and thoughts. Make sure you don't let things like your shopping list slip in there – it's a private and personal record of your feelings, hopes and fears, and you don't want to trivialise it by mixing it up with the minutiae of domestic life. If you are more comfortable writing online, you may like to use a free and secure journal such as penzu.com – anything that allows you to be thoroughly honest with yourself.

Try not to write too self-consciously, as the inner censor is a powerful force and will use any excuse to mask your real feelings. Keep it somewhere you know nobody else will see it, and allow yourself to really let go. It doesn't matter if your sentences are misspelt or ungrammatical, or whether you just write, 'I hate the world, it's not fair', over and over again at the beginning. What you do with it is totally up to you. And remember, just because you've written something down doesn't mean it will stay like that for ever. You may feel angry and resentful towards your partner one day, but try not to feel guilty when, the following week, everything seems fine. Feelings are just feelings – they change regularly and writing them down in a safe place is a good way of getting them out of your system. Feeling is something you *do*, not something you *are*. Often, the simple act of writing down a thought that has been obsessively whirling about in your head is enough to remove its power over you.

I find it helpful to write first thing in the morning, before my inner censor has had a chance to get to work, but for some people that's not convenient, so find a time that suits you. The most important thing is that you write something every day. Some people like to re-read what they've written, others just want to use it as a place to dump obsessive thoughts and move on.

The 80/20 rule

A good way to use the journal is as part of the 80/20 rule. I believe that when there's something big and stressful happening in your life, it's totally unrealistic to expect that you should ignore it or put it to the back of your mind. One way to regain a feeling of control in your life is to focus intensely on your worry for 20% of your time, and let it go (to the best of your ability) for the other 80%. So, for you, the 20% might include writing in your journal, doing some research on the Internet, calling a support line, making an appointment with an alternative therapist – anything that focuses entirely on your fertility. And then try to let go. Experiencing infertility can sometimes feel like you're holding your breath for six months, a year, six years – however long it's been – and I find it helpful to focus on learning techniques and strategies that will help you to let go of that breath and rediscover a sense of yourself in the here and now.

The gratitude list

Another useful tool is a gratitude list. You might not feel like being grateful for anything right now, but it can be really helpful to acknowledge the good things that you *do* have in your life.

Do you have a partner helping you through the process? A supportive family and/or friends? Good health generally? Fulfilling work? A well-developed sense of the absurd? Maybe you're just grateful you have a roof over your head and that you live in a free country. Or that you can look out of your window each morning and appreciate the birdsong around you, and the beauty of your urban or rural environment. The level to which you go is entirely up to you; what matters is that you recognise that there are positive things in your life, and that you're not just a host for malfunctioning ovaries, or whatever your problem is.

Try to write down three new things each morning and acknowledge that, despite the sadness and frustration you may be feeling, there is also room for other, positive emotions. It won't devalue or belittle your desire for a baby, but it can help you regain a sense of perspective. It's a discipline and it can sometimes feel really hard – especially when you've just gone through a cycle that hasn't worked, or the lab has come back with some disappointing test results. But the more you do it, the more it helps – I promise you.

Nutrition and alternative therapies

There are many fantastic resources available to support you during your fertility treatment, and this book is intended to complement, not replace, them. To that end, you won't find a chapter here on what you should eat, or whether you should have acupuncture, reflexology, reiki, or any other treatment that you have heard might help. At the back of this book, there are links to organisations, books and websites that have helped me and my clients, and it's up to you if you choose to try them out for yourself. Many people find that following a particular therapy has been useful for them, but if you're already sceptical about such treatments, I'd advise you to approach with caution. Nothing will *guarantee* you getting pregnant – it's about finding an approach that works for you. And if you find yourself spending all your money on a series of alternative therapies, you could end up resenting the outlay and exceeding the 80/20 rule, despite your best intentions. Also, while there are treatments and resources that have helped me and others, they are by no means essential to achieving a successful pregnancy, and you should not worry if you don't have the money to spend on additional therapies.

Many of my clients are intensely focused on their bodies. It shows in their posture – they have come to see themselves as a series of symptoms and problems. My role is to help them understand the mind/body connection. Often, people are so focused on their condition that they lose sight of who they are. The aim of this book is to help you regain a sense of yourself and a holistic idea of the real you, aside from your fertility issues.

Humour

No – I'm not joking. It might seem on the surface that there's no place for laughter in a book on a subject as difficult as infertility. You may feel right now as if you'll never laugh again. But you will, and it can actually be a powerful weapon in your struggle. A well-known blogger in the world of fertility, Infertile Naomi, has come up with 999 reasons to laugh at infertility,[2] and the feedback on her website and Facebook page testifies to the support she has given to women worldwide. I'm not going to cite all 999 reasons, but here are a few ideas that made me smile:

- Buy a darker shade of toilet paper. Be honest: you spend most of your time inspecting the toilet paper for signs of ovulation, indications of your period or implantation bleeding. Even when you try not to look, you still do. Buy a darker shade of paper so you can't see when the blood has arrived. Or, at least, buy toilet paper in bulk.
- Keep an emergency 'I just got my period' kit on hand. Getting your period or doing a negative pregnancy test can bring days of heartache and despair, so stock up on things you love. Your kit might include a bottle of wine, chocolate, bath soap or anything else that makes you happy.
- Don't succumb to infertility amnesia. An infertility amnesiac is someone who obsesses about fertility and wanting a baby on

a daily basis, and forgets how blessed they already are. They ignore the fact that they have a wonderful family, great friends and a healthy body and mind. The good news is, there is a cure for infertility amnesia, but it starts with you.

■ Give yourself the 10-minute cry. When you have a negative pregnancy test allow yourself to cry for no more than 10 minutes. Continuing to cry all month means a lot of wasted tears and energy. In that 10 minutes, feel sorry for yourself and have a really good cry – one with lots of tears, swollen eyes and a runny nose. After 10 minutes, breathe and move on.

■ Laugh at yourself. Whether we want to admit it or not, we do a lot of strange things in order to get pregnant. Next time you are inspecting the toilet paper, or analysing your breasts for early signs of pregnancy take a moment to smile. Happiness is a choice, and from infertility can come strength.

■ Oh – and my favourite: you know you're infertile when ... your boss asks you what day it is, and you respond: 'Day 15.'

The part humour can play in successful IVF treatment has been studied. In Israel, a doctor hired his friend, a chef and clown, to visit patients after embryo transfer. He performed magic tricks and told jokes about his experiences in the kitchen (presumably without too many references to eggs). Two groups were observed: 93 women who didn't watch the clown and 93 who did. The first group had a 19% success rate. Amazingly, 35% of the second group became pregnant. I kid you not.

The key here is to be proactive. Seek out the people and things that naturally make you laugh – specific friends, films, books, pets – and fill your life with them. Try to look for moments of the absurd even in the midst of your quest to get pregnant. At one point, I remember laughing till I cried with my husband at the lengths to which we were going in order to conceive: acupuncture, hypnotherapy, zinc bangles, coaching, nutritional advice, prayer, and the final straw for him: taking an expensive tree bark supplement in order to improve his sperm quality. How did we get here, we asked each other, and then started laughing uncontrollably. It was a great moment. If you can find humour even in the darkness, the journey will become so much easier.

CHAPTER 2

MAKE CONNECTIONS: LINKING MIND AND BODY

"If you do what you've always done, you'll get what you've always got."
Mark Twain

What are you thinking right now? If you stop and listen to your thoughts for a second, what can you hear? What kind of script can you see in your mind's eye? So many of us go through the day (and sometimes the whole night) with the same words buzzing round our minds, blissfully unaware of the impact that this 'self-talk' is having on our lives.

Scientists, philosophers and healers throughout the centuries have understood the close relationship between what goes on in our heads and what happens to our bodies. More recently, doctors and psychologists have been looking at the effect of the way we think on our ability to conceive, particularly with IVF treatment.

A recent study[1] by doctors at Soroka Medical Center in Beersheba, Israel, looked into the impact of hypnosis on 185 women undergoing IVF. It found that 28% of the women who had been hypnotised became pregnant, compared to just 14% who had not.

Another study[2] by researchers at Emory University in Atlanta provided strong evidence of the success of cognitive behavioural therapy (CBT) in treating women who were having trouble ovulating.

They discovered that, of the women who had CBT, 75% recovered full fertility whereas only 12.5% did so without the treatment.

Other studies, too numerous to mention here, demonstrate the links between stress and depression and difficulty in conceiving. Dr Alice Domar,[3] a world-renowned expert on infertility and the author of many useful books on the subject, also undertook a number of research projects at the Domar Center for Mind/Body Health in Boston and concluded: 'Mind/body treatment has been shown to be effective in both significantly increasing pregnancy rates as well as reducing psychological stress.'

I would like to point out here that, while reducing stress and gaining a sense of control over your thoughts and behaviour will not guarantee a pregnancy, it could increase your chances. I'm sure you could find plenty of examples out there of women who have conceived during periods of intense stress or bereavement. In fact, you may already have come across people who will tell you that acupuncture/good nutrition/regular exercise made no difference in their case ('I ate nothing but Mars bars and worked 18-hour days, and had no trouble getting pregnant') but that's about them – or their friend, or sister, or whoever else they're using to back up their theory.

All I can say is that there is a wealth of research showing that hormone levels, ovulation and other reproductive factors may well be affected by what's going on in your head. And if you're having trouble conceiving, it makes sense to give yourself the best possible chances of success – with what's in your control, at least.

I trained and practised for a number of years as a coach with Powerchange, an organisation run by a wonderful and inspiring man called Andrew Sercombe, who changes the life of everyone he meets. I am grateful that he has given me permission to share with you some of the tools he created to help change the way we think and behave. Here is one of my favourites.

Powerchange tool: DASA

This is a highly effective exercise for helping you to find out what you want – and then helping you to get it. DASA stands for: **D**ecide what you want; **A**ct towards it; **S**ee what happens; **A**djust. But before you decide what you want, it helps to truly understand the mind/body connection. Change your mind and your body will follow. Walk boldly and you will start to think boldly. Thought is your body in action, the process of your brain cells at work. What happens in one changes the other. Notice the mind/body connection when:

- You are talking to others
- You are talking to yourself
- You are listening to yourself
- You are watching others as you listen to them, and as you talk to them

It can help to write down these thoughts as you become increasingly aware of them. There's no need to censor or react to what you are saying, just note them down as they appear. When you have a few pages of the 'evidence' of your conversations with yourself and others, ask yourself:

- What is the pattern to my thoughts and words?
- What is the general theme? Is it positive or negative, healthy or destructive?
- Knowing what you do about the power of thoughts to influence the body, are these the kind of thoughts and words you would choose in order to be living the sort of life you want?
- If so, congratulations – keep at it. If not, what kind of thoughts or words might you choose to replace the others in order to better influence your body?

Decide what you want

Having a clear idea of what you want forces the brain to move strongly in that direction. By defining in your imagination as fully as possible what you are aiming for, you will find that your brain will work away at the project, even when you're asleep. It is important to put your goal into a positive framework, as the brain tends not to process negatives. So, if you say, 'I don't want to be overweight', your brain will just hear 'be overweight' and it will be harder to achieve your goal. With this example, you might want to replace it with, 'I want to be slim and healthy.'

For some people, having their own baby is the only thing they want at this stage. Ask: 'When I have that, what will it give me?' Others discover that what they want is a sense of peace and fulfillment, whatever the outcome.

I try to encourage my clients to explore the concept of 'family' in the widest sense, as there is more than one way to achieve it, and being open to the greater meaning of the word can unearth previously unconsidered possibilities. Allow a little flexibility when you're setting your goals. That doesn't mean don't go for what you want. It's just that being flexible and investigating 'greater' goals than you thought possible will actually help you to achieve what you want – as well as other positive outcomes you couldn't initially have imagined. Flexibility is empowering.

Act towards it

Act towards the outcome you have identified. Deliberately do something that will change the present circumstances in favour of your goal. The problem for many people is that they want to do the 'right thing' when there isn't a single 'right thing' to do – there are hundreds of possible 'right' options. The wrong thing is definitely to do nothing.

Acting towards your outcome:
- Shows your unconscious mind you mean business;
- Gives your unconscious mind your permission and authority to get to work on the desired outcome;
- Demonstrates your physical commitment and actually starts the external process.

Ask yourself, 'What can I do that will make things happen?' When I went through my own DASA process, I found that 'acting towards it' meant lots of research on the Internet, because for me, the more information I have at my disposal, the more in control I feel. But you may feel differently, and your 'acting towards it' could involve taking yourself off for a weekend break to get some distance from your situation and connect with your partner in the great outdoors.

One of my clients had been through two-and-a-half cycles of IVF and came to the conclusion that two of her options were as diverse as deciding to accept donated eggs, or spending the £7,000 she would otherwise have invested in her treatment on the holiday of a lifetime. Your options may not be as extreme as hers, but the more you can do in order to achieve your desired outcome, the freer you will feel.

A word of warning: most people undergoing fertility treatment are part of a couple and you also need to think about your partner's feelings. Even if you both agree about the process, you will need to go at the pace of the 'slower' individual. And by this, I don't mean physically or intellectually slow. People are willing to look at different options at different speeds and, although it may be frustrating initially, it is important for your relationship that you both travel at the same pace to meet your goals. This can mean that you might need to wait a while if, for example, you have decided that surrogacy or adoption would be a viable option, but your partner isn't there yet. There are too many instances of couples splitting up when one was actively pursuing an avenue of treatment that the other wasn't ready to deal with.

See what happens

We use 'see' here in the wider sense of 'notice the changes that result from your new behaviour'. This is probably the most neglected element of DASA. Look carefully at what happened when you acted. What changed? Is this what you had in mind?

'Seeing what happens' may not be quite what you think. It doesn't involve just sitting with your feet up, passively waiting for a miracle. It is the 'seeing what happens' that a research scientist does. Keep looking for the little tell-tale signs of change. Internal changes can mean you see things differently, you feel different, your self-talk has changed. External changes can be seen in the world around you, in your body and in your interactions with other people.

During this period, you may experience huge changes or, indeed, discover that the actions you hoped would produce change didn't, in which case you are now one step nearer to your goal by eliminating something that doesn't work. In either case, you are likely to be experiencing a wide range of emotions, some of which may be unfamiliar to you. It is important in these situations to have an outlet in addition to your partner for offloading and releasing your feelings. Although it is vital that you keep the channels of communication with your partner open and tell them regularly how you feel, it can be a bit overwhelming for them to be the sole repository of your emotions. It's crucial to have conversations with your partner that are totally unconnected to your fertility issues or babies in general – it's what will remind you of why you want a family with this person, and give you some perspective on your issues. So, make sure you have a number of friends you can speak to, join a support group, call a helpline, or go online to one of the fertility chat rooms if you find them helpful. You can also use your journal for recording your feelings about the DASA process.

Adjust

The final step in DASA is to adjust, whether internally or externally, to help you move towards that end goal of family.

- How flexible are you?
- What new ways of 'being yourself' are you ready to learn?

The three-question technique

My clients come to me with a variety of issues, but one thing they often have in common is a mindset that they have taken on after looking at the evidence they have about their situation and drawing conclusions from it. Unfortunately, however, the conclusion may bear little resemblance to objective reality as you or I might see it. Yes, we do all see things differently and subjectively, but sometimes our take on our circumstances might not be helping us – or our partner, family or friends.

When I come across a limiting belief (you can usually spot these a mile off from the use of generalisations, or vague but negative statements presented as fact), I like to challenge it with the following questions:

- Is this statement true?
- Is it helpful for me?
- Is it helpful for anyone else?

One client of mine had experienced two failed IVF cycles and came to me to discuss the next stage as she saw it – adoption. But while I was talking to her, it became apparent that her beliefs were based solely on those two failed cycles. Her limiting belief drawn from this 'evidence' was: 'My body's not working.'

While it might have been the case that adoption was the most appropriate route further down the line, I felt that she was making a huge generalisation about her biology without sufficient information to back it up. If she chose to explore adoption, it should be because this was the best of all the options available to her. So, in this instance, the most important question for her to answer was: 'Is this statement true?'

She went back to the clinic and asked for feedback about the process, and discovered that, although the cycles hadn't been successful, there was nothing specifically wrong with the embryos and no reason why another attempt wouldn't work. (Incidentally, I have found that it's definitely worth being proactive in getting information from your clinic. They may not always give you as much detail as you would like, however, so make sure you ask everything that's on your mind, to satisfy yourself you know as much as possible about the process.)

So, the statement wasn't objectively true: her body was working. Was it helpful for her? Not particularly, as it left her with only one possible option as far as she was concerned and, therefore, she wasn't making a real choice. Was it helpful for anyone else? For the same reasons, probably not.

Sometimes our negative self-talk isn't really ours at all. We may be thinking the thoughts, but the voices in our head can be those of family members or other authority figures from our childhood. Even offhand comments with no real malice behind them can stay lodged in our heads for years and seriously affect the way we think and feel about ourselves. In coaching, we call these 'limiting beliefs', because they stop us from achieving our true potential. At worst, they can keep us in unsatisfying jobs or bad relationships and make us truly miserable. They are the enemies of a happy and fulfilling life.

Exercise: unearthing limiting beliefs

It can take a bit of practice to unearth all your limiting beliefs – but digging them out and examining them under the microscope can be one of the most liberating things you've ever done. The trick is to catch yourself in the midst of thinking those limiting thoughts and to write them down.

One way of identifying them is to draw up a number of lists. On one, write: 'Five things my mother said about me were...', and repeat for your father, your grandparents, your teachers – anyone who had any influence on your young life. It may surprise you to discover that you have internalised a significant number of negative beliefs – and these are a great place to start with the three-question technique. What myths about yourself or the world can you explode right now?

CASE STUDY

Being willing to examine your thoughts and beliefs and respond with action can take a lot of courage, but it will pay off many times over. Meet Sarah, a courageous former client of mine who is living a happier life today as a result of transforming her negative thinking.

SARAH'S STORY

Getting the diagnosis of polycystic ovary syndrome (PCOS) was a bit of a shock as I'd had none of the symptoms you'd normally associate with the condition - excess weight, facial hair, acne. I'd been taking the pill for several years and my cycles had been normal before that, so the pill must have masked the development of the condition over time.

We'd been trying for a baby for less than a year, but I was really struggling to come to terms with the diagnosis, and I needed some support to help with my feelings. My friends tried to understand, but they'd say things like, 'It'll happen eventually' or 'Just relax, it'll happen' - well-meaning but totally unhelpful. So I decided to get some coaching as I wanted to speak to someone who understood and I didn't know anyone else in my situation. I did talk to my husband, but it was difficult to discuss certain things because I was worried about upsetting him.

I had a lot of guilt about my feelings, and would often feel bad about avoiding social situations where there would be a lot of pregnant women, but I gradually learnt to be kinder to myself. It was almost as if I needed permission to stop pushing myself so hard and trying to be perfect.

I got a lot better at being kind to myself. I'd led quite a busy life, commuting into London, but I decided to leave my job as a chartered accountant to become a primary school teacher, which is what I'd been doing several years before. It was closer to home – less commuting, less stress. A positive move.

I really worked on myself mentally and physically – I did acupuncture and reflexology and followed the Foresight method [a programme that advises couples on nutrition, health, allergies, etc]. I had had six rounds of [the fertility drug] Clomid before this, which helped to restore my cycles, but we wanted to try alternative therapies before putting ourselves on the IVF waiting list. I used the three-question technique a lot, as I had a real tendency to think negatively, and talked through other difficult stuff in my past that had come up during the coaching sessions. I also tried to think of three good things each day that I had in my life. It did make me feel better to focus on my husband or my friends or even my house.

I think being less negative also made things easier for my husband. I went through phases where I'd say to him, 'You should go off and find someone else who doesn't have these problems', and in hindsight, it was hard and emotionally draining for him to keep reassuring me. And when I stopped blaming myself and started looking after myself more, that also took the strain off him.

I got pregnant naturally in October 2009 – so whether it was the coaching, the reflexology, the acupuncture, the nutrition or the career change, something helped it happen. And my attitude towards myself has definitely changed: I now know I'm worth looking after.

CHAPTER 3

TO THYSELF BE TRUE: BEING YOU

"Talents are best nurtured in solitude, but character is best formed in the stormy billows of the world."
Johann Wolfgang von Goethe

Who are you? If you're embarking on, or are in the middle of, having fertility treatment right now, it might not be such an easy question to answer. However, a strong and grounded sense of who you are is perhaps one of the most important elements in helping you to stay sane throughout the process.

Our lives today so often seem to be centred on what we do, or the things we have. When we meet someone at a party, for example, one of the first questions we ask them is: 'What do you do?' Our occupation tends to define us, and we describe ourselves in the same way: 'I'm a teacher', or 'I work for a bank', or, as we often hear, 'I'm just a housewife' – as if our lack of paid employment makes us somehow 'less than'. We may also focus on what we have as a way to define our happiness, or lack of it. So many people 'create' an identity by wearing clothes by a particular designer or buying a certain make of car that they feel helps them to belong. But that's getting things the wrong way round. We need to *be* who we are in order to *do* what we need to do to *have* what we want. Trying to be a certain person through the work we do or the products we buy may feel like it is working for a while. But it will only ever be temporary, and trying to create an identity this way round will be more likely to make you feel empty and unfulfilled in the long term.

I'm not saying that the work you do isn't tremendously important, and a vital part of your wellbeing and fulfilment. Stimulating and challenging employment can be one of life's great joys. But it's not *who* you are, it's a *part* of it. You may know someone who lives for their work but struggles to hold a conversation about anything outside their field of interest. In the same way, it's important to do what you can to prevent yourself obsessing about your treatment or having a child.

You may feel I'm asking you to do the impossible, but it is vital to broaden your thoughts and activities, not only for your own sake, but also for that of your family, friends and partner. You'll need their support more than ever now, but you're more likely to receive it if they feel they are engaging with the person they've always known and loved. It may seem an obvious point, but try to be aware of how much you talk about your issues, and to whom. You are more than your current problems. You're the person your partner fell in love with, the person your best friend went out dancing with, the person who sat next to them on the first day of school. It's so important to remember what you mean to those around you, and to nurture the close relationships that will sustain you throughout your life.

A changing sense of self

Fertility issues inevitably impact on your sense of self – but many of us don't realise to what extent until we're in the middle of an identity crisis. Liz Scott, a counsellor at the Lister Fertility Clinic in London, says that many of her clients are typically high achievers who have worked hard in their lives and been rewarded by obtaining their goals throughout their education and career. 'This may be the first time they no longer feel in control of their life as they recognise that, no matter how much money, emotional or physical energy they invest in treatment, they cannot guarantee a positive outcome,' she explains. Often, she sees identity issues come up when others in their peer group or family achieve what they desire most – a child of their own. Liz says:

'Many women no longer feel they hold the same position in their peer group or society because of their inability to have a child, and may feel excluded from groups of friends who now meet as families, together with their children. As women feel less confident and less in control, they become more anxious and stressed, and it is often at this point that they will seek counselling.'

The key word here is 'control'. As Liz points out: 'While you may not have control over the outcome of the process, you *do* have control over how you manage it' – and this involves maintaining and developing your identity outside of your fertility problems.

Three key words

This is a quick, fun exercise to find out how your friends and family see you – with the added benefit of reminding them that you are more than your current issues. If they had to define you using just three adjectives, which ones would they choose? Ask as many people as you trust – you might be surprised by the variety of responses. Make sure you write them down in your journal. Once you have asked five people, you will have 15 words that describe you – and I bet none of them is 'infertile'.

One of my clients came to me saying she felt low because she'd been so wrapped up in her treatment, she wasn't being a good enough friend – something that was clearly an important part of the way she viewed herself. We worked with the three-question technique described in Chapter 2 to find out if there was any truth to her statement. It turned out that she was still seeing her friends quite a lot – but there were a few 'high-maintenance' people whom she had always supported in the past who wanted more from her than she was currently able to give. She concluded that, for the time being, she would focus on the friendships that were more reciprocal, in which she didn't feel she needed to give more than she got. I also asked her to include some of the more 'equal' friends in her three key words investigation and, as it turned out, several of them included 'good friend' as one of the defining descriptions.

Personal ad

Another variation on the three key words exercise is for you to write a personal ad, such as those you might see in the newspapers' 'soul-mates' columns. Try to keep it to less than 100 words, but include all the important points about you – and keep it truthful. What really interests you? What makes you tick? What are your most appealing characteristics? If you're feeling really brave, you could show this to a friend or your partner to see what they would add, but that's not essential for the exercise to work. Put it aside and then reread it the following day, when you've got a bit of distance. What do you think of the person described in the ad? It's you. Well, if you've been truthful, it's the bits of you that might not have been exposed for a while. How could you incorporate the 'fun-loving', 'adventurous' or 'passionate about music' parts of your character into your life today? What three things could you do this week to awaken those dormant parts of your soul?

Of course, you're not going to feel 'fun-loving' or 'adventurous' every day. We're all human, and have good days as well as bad. Many of my clients are used to success in their working lives and 'making things happen'; they start panicking when they have a bad day, and none of their coping strategies seems to be hitting the spot. On days like these, when you don't want to get out of bed, let alone confide in a friend, it's important to be kind to yourself. One of the more damaging aspects of modern life is the expectation that, as long as you look good and read the right books and 'do the right thing', everything will be fine. It's usually the companies with a vested commercial interest in our unhappiness that propagate this notion, but nonetheless it can be damaging if left unchallenged.

When we experience periods of extreme stress, we go through a series of emotions – and we tend to label the ones we feel comfortable with as 'good' and anything else that seems irrational or unkind as 'bad'. The fact is, we are whole human beings with a variety of feelings, and it is critical for our emotional health to give ourselves permission to experience them all. That doesn't mean we abdicate all responsibility for how we choose to act on them, but denying our 'dark side' can be as damaging as acting on it too much. Some of us were brought up to believe that if we had 'bad thoughts', we would be punished, either by an adult or by some all-seeing deity. Suppressing parts of ourselves can mean that we end up acting out the very behaviour we are seeking to avoid – or it may come out in a different way.

For example, if we are angry with our partner but don't feel safe acknowledging that (maybe we don't think there's a good enough reason, or it would be unkind), our feelings may slip out in other ways – through sarcasm, passive–aggressive behaviour or by overreacting to a comment. The safest way to deal with feelings like this is to write them down in your journal. Just thinking something doesn't make you a bad person. Often, the act of writing something down helps you see your options more clearly, and you can choose to act in a way that is congruous with your values. This underlines the need to keep your journal completely private, though. If you feel angry after speaking to a good friend who has just told you she's pregnant, or you're terrified your partner will leave you if your treatment is not successful, write it down. It doesn't matter if it 'doesn't make sense': what's important is accepting yourself and your feelings – not just the 'acceptable' ones – as a whole.

The fact is, you are worth exactly the same, whatever thoughts you might have had, or things you might have said. Let me put that another way – your worth is not contingent upon variables such as your past, your actions, or your thoughts, in the same way that it doesn't depend on your skin colour, where you were born or what you believe. Of course, you have values and morals that shape how you act and the way you want to be. But as a human being, you have the same worth as anyone else – what you choose to do with that humanity is another issue.

So, it's natural to want to do things right and be happy – I believe that is an understandable human impulse. But it's worth remembering when you're having a bad day that although your feelings might be different, you are still you. And that person is priceless.

One of my clients had a ring inscribed with 'This too shall pass', for when the bad days got her down. When I was going through what seemed like my hundredth IVF cycle, I felt that the experience would make me or break me as a person, and I was determined that it would be the former. Before I began my treatment, I had a huge phobia of needles, as well as general anaesthetic. One evening, as I was injecting myself in the stomach with a blood-thinning drug for the thirty-second week in a row, I realised how far I'd come. It was a real moment of revelation for me, to discover that I was now automatically doing what I had never thought I could. I felt so proud of myself that I wrote it down in my journal, as a reminder for when I had bad days of just what I'd achieved.

Exercise

- How often do you have bad days? What kind of thoughts go through your head? What happens? Describe them as fully as you can.
- What could you do to help you cope on those days? They don't have to be big things. It could be buying your favourite food or calling a friend you don't need to be 'up' for. How many ways can you think of of being kind to yourself?
- What experiences have you been through in the past that have contributed to you becoming the person you are today? What are you most proud of?
- Try to get into the habit of writing down three things each day for which you can be proud of yourself. Did you bite your tongue when your mother-in-law asked when she could expect a grandchild? Did you say 'no' to a social function because you were feeling tired and needed to look after yourself? Acknowledge them all.

Lose yourself

What do you really love doing? What causes you to lose track of time because you're concentrating hard and enjoying the moment? For me, it's singing. I may not be the world's best singer, but I can honestly say that I never feel more myself than when I'm belting out a tune, whether in the privacy of my own home or in company. For some people it's playing chess, for others it's painting or cooking or running. Most of us have something that makes us feel 'in the zone' – and there's nothing more life-affirming than indulging that instinct and going with the flow to help you exist in the present. If you haven't got a 'thing' – experiment. Make it a personal project to discover what it is that makes you feel alive, and then do it.

Powerchange tool: creating an attractive future

This is a fantastic exercise that has helped my clients focus on their identity and their future in a holistic, motivating way.

Who you are

- Describe three aspects of your character – who you are – that you are proud of.
- What sort of person do you want to be? Focus on character. Express your thoughts in your own words and note any particular areas for improvement.
- If someone were asked to sum up your life with an epitaph, what might it say? What would you like it to say?
- Choose one aspect of your character you would like to improve. How will being this way benefit you and others in the future?

Little in life is free. We usually have to pay for what we get – and get what we pay for. Considering your time, energy, money, words, reputation, creative thoughts, ethics, choice of friends, attitudes and anything else that comes to mind:

- List two significant things you are prepared to exchange for what you want.
- List two significant things you will not, under any circumstances, exchange.

What you do

- Summarise what you have achieved through your own effort, actions and commitment - professional or personal. Include things you're proud of as well as things you aren't.

Your wish list

- What do you wish, secretly or otherwise, you had done in the past few years? As with the other exercises, it will be most helpful if you can focus on things you have control over in your life, rather than just your fertility journey.
- Give your reasons for any differences between what you have actually done and what you wish you had done.
- What desire is currently outstanding that you believe to be achievable and within your control?
- What resources do you need to achieve this?
- Where are those resources and how can you access them?
- Comment on how your behaviour has affected other people in the past.
- How is it currently affecting other people?
- How has it affected your own success?

CHAPTER 4

GET GOING! TIME TO ACT

"We are what we repeatedly do."
Aristotle

I'm a doer – albeit one guilty of sometimes thinking too much. But when I have a problem or I'm feeling unhappy, my first instinct is to react immediately. What can I do to change this situation, make it better, feel more comfortable? This was never more apparent than when I was waiting for those pregnancy-test results two weeks after egg transfer. It's all too easy for people to try to persuade you to adopt a Zen attitude of inner peace and tranquillity, but we're only human and the treatment process can push your patience to its limits.

For those who feel the need to act, I have some good news – there are many things you can do to take control during this frustrating time. Admittedly, you can't make that embryo implant (if only), but it is possible to hold onto your sanity if, like me, you feel that action is what keeps you going.

A word here on how activity and identity fit together; after reading Chapter 3 on the importance of *being*, it would be understandable if you were a little confused about the focus here on *doing*. But they're not mutually exclusive – they are truly interdependent. Your identity and value are part of the 'you' at the core of your being. But humans are creatures of habit, and our activities go a long way towards shaping who we are. We can find ourselves in dangerous territory if we concentrate on *doing* to the exclusion of everything else. As

I mentioned before, it can be tempting to define ourselves by our success in our professional lives, and let our 'work doing' represent who we are. During fertility treatment, we need to focus on a new type of doing, one that will enhance our feeling of control without becoming obsessive. I used to make lists during the difficult times. A typical weekend day might have included:

- Write in my journal for half an hour
- Make an appointment with the acupuncturist
- Spend half an hour on an Internet fertility forum
- Read a book on nutrition
- Go for coffee with a friend
- Book tickets for a concert in a few months' time

And so on. In some ways, the content of what I did mattered less than knowing that I was doing *everything within my power* to influence a positive result and retain my identity as Anya Sizer. And that, ironically, made it easier to let go of what was out of my control. I also found it important when focusing on 'actions' to look at my future life in the widest possible sense.

A popular coaching tool that my clients have found invaluable when trying to achieve a balance between being and doing, is the wheel of life. It's a great way to visually represent how you spend your time, and can motivate you to make changes in certain areas that words alone might not have identified.

Wheel of life

- Choose six different and important aspects of your life. These could be job/career, family, social life, play and fun, spirituality, health, learning, eating, sleeping, goal-setting, etc – whatever you feel is important.

- Write one choice on each spoke of the wheel.
- With zero being the centre of the wheel and the outer rim representing your ideal amount of attention, mark where you currently are and join up the dots.

Wheel of Life

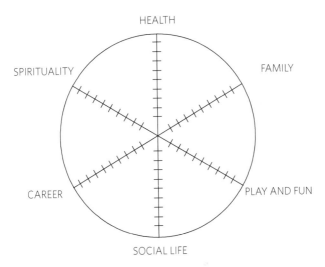

Wheel of life is a tool to help a person gain an overview of their life at the present time and to from there look at ways to move on.

The middle point is represented by a 0 and the outer rim by a 10, the person allocates a score for each one.

When I was going through infertility I probably would have scored it thus:

CAREER	4	FAMILY	4
SOCIAL LIFE	6	PLAY AND FUN	5
SPIRITUALITY	7	HEALTH	8

- What does this exercise highlight for you?
- How can/will you create solutions to this situation?
- What changes do you want to make to the balance of the wheel?
- What time frame do you have for this?

When I look back at the diaries I wrote while going through IVF, I see a lot of confusion and anxiety, but also a determination to live my life to the full, regardless of my situation. During so much of this process, you feel like you're underwater, holding your breath. I knew I couldn't make time move any faster, but it certainly felt like it did if my days were full.

One 'doing' thing that helped was being consciously altruistic. Fertility treatment makes you hyper-aware of your body and mind, and it can feel like you're constantly watching yourself for signs of possible pregnancy. Self-awareness is a good thing (especially when it comes to feelings), but sometimes it can be beneficial to focus on others, as it gives you a bit of perspective on your situation, as well as enhancing your wellbeing, ironically enough. There have been various studies to show how volunteering improves both physical and mental health[1] – as well as helping others, of course. We chose to sponsor a child overseas during our treatment, but there are plenty of things you could do, including:

- Helping an elderly neighbour with the shopping
- Getting out into the fresh air and volunteering on a conservation project
- Reading with a primary-school child at lunchtime
- Coaching a local sports team at the weekend
- Creating posters or leaflets for a local charity

If you are based in the UK, you can visit your local Volunteer Centre for information about activities in your area (see the online resources at the back of this book for more details). The possibilities are endless, but be aware of how you are feeling if you choose to volunteer with young children. I remember finding it hard to spend time with visibly pregnant women when I felt low. It may be fine for you, but just monitor your mood and look after yourself.

I also found it useful to read a newspaper regularly to keep up with what was going on in the world around me – not out of a sense of guilt, or to beat myself up that there were 'other people worse off than me' (although that doesn't hurt), but to feel connected to my surroundings. It's easy to let your world shrink as you focus on your treatment and your body, and finding ways to reach out can make you feel healthier – and saner.

Here are some more tips from my clients and fertility support-group members who were willing to share their experiences of what worked for them. Not everything will be appropriate for your situation, but sometimes the smallest things can make a big difference to your mental health:

- Find a good support group.
- Don't fret if your friends 'don't get' how you feel, but reach out to new ones who do.
- Do something fun just for you at least once a week. You may not be able to relax on command, but you can pamper yourself every now and then.
- Destress with meditation, hypnotherapy or acupuncture.
- Find a therapist. Mine came via the NHS (from a GP referral) and was fantastic.
- Research your particular condition or issue on reputable websites and do everything you can (diet, herbal remedies, etc.) to help yourself regain control.
- Plan little things to look forward to on a regular basis – a meal out, a country walk or a concert – so there are positives as well as all the difficulties.

CASE STUDY

Alison, 42, is one of my former clients. She and her husband had been trying to conceive for nearly three years before seeing a consultant, who diagnosed a hydrosalpinx (a type of blockage) on her right fallopian tube and recommended they start fertility treatment. I asked her if she would be willing to share her story to demonstrate how taking control of your situation and being aware of your thoughts really can make a difference.

ALISON'S STORY

To complement my fertility treatment, I decided to see a nutritionist and an acupuncturist, to ensure I was doing all I could. If it failed this time, I didn't want to look back and say: 'I wish I'd tried that.' That's when I decided to have some coaching as well, to prepare myself mentally. What immediately helped was realising the impact of how I talked to myself – and being made aware that there were a lot of negative words in my vocabulary that I needed to eliminate. Other exercises I learnt that were really beneficial were the wheel of life and the three-question technique.

The main thing that made a difference, though, was being able to talk to someone who'd been there and knew what I was going through – especially during the two-week wait after egg transfer. It was good to be able to call or email to ask 'Is this normal?' I also found visualisation helpful – imagining how I wanted things to turn out – and that's a tool I've used since the treatment in other areas of my life.

I did go and see a counsellor at the clinic once, but they immediately started talking about adoption, and I thought: 'Adoption? I don't want to hear this.' I wasn't ready to think about it then.

I am lucky to have such a close and supportive relationship with my husband and family – it's so important, as the whole process is an emotional rollercoaster and can put your marriage to the test. The treatment is very much centred on the woman, and the men seem to get left out of the process. It's a stressful time and my husband only had me to support him, but you get so wrapped up in your own feelings, you can forget what they may be going through.

There are a few things I wish I'd known before my treatment – for example, it can take several attempts to become pregnant, although there are some women who are lucky enough to conceive the first time with IVF. I also think you can read too much. It's finding a balance between doing as much as you can to help yourself, and going overboard. You need to feel relaxed, so a glass of wine always helps. When I finally did get pregnant with IVF, I was advised by a private midwife not to do any exercise (except walking) for the first 12 weeks, so I wrapped myself up in cotton wool: I was afraid I would lose the baby if I exerted myself. I think it's common for women who've had treatment to worry more – those who get pregnant naturally don't seem to stress as much – but I wish I'd not been so anxious.

We are very, very lucky that we ended up with such a beautiful little girl. She's a really special baby.

Powerchange tool: the now audit

One technique that has served me well, both during treatment and in the course of my everyday life, is making sure I'm aware of my priorities. Modern life places increasing demands on us all, and you can find yourself overwhelmed with activities and commitments because you're not entirely sure what your limits are, both physically and emotionally. I find going through a quick 'now audit' a great way to bring myself back into the present and relax, sure about what I need to commit to – and certain what belongs in the past, or the future. In your journal:

- Write down everything that has significance for you. This can be material items, or it can be feelings or attitudes. So, for example, your list could include: my car; half of the mortgage on my flat; my behaviour towards my partner; my memories; my health, etc.
- Make sure you record only what is here in the present.
- If you're not sure whether to include something on the list, write it down anyway, but make sure that if it's a joint responsibility (such as your house or bringing up your children) you acknowledge your share of it. Don't take responsibility for items that should be on someone else's list.
- When your list is finished, you will have in front of you the sum total of your responsibilities, no more, no less. Although it may be different tomorrow, this is what you have now. The rest is speculation and imagination.
- Now, go through your list and allocate a score from 0 to 10 (where 0 is the least demanding) to each item, in answer to the question: 'How demanding is this?'

- Look at each high-scoring item and ask yourself: 'What decision needs to be made about this?' Anything with a very high score is likely to be the source of stress (or neglect) and require action.
- Record your decision, along with a date and time when you plan to act on it. Hold yourself accountable and do it.

CHAPTER 5

CHART YOUR JOURNEY: MAKE TIME WORK FOR YOU

"Make use of time, let not advantage slip."
William Shakespeare

When you're trying to conceive, everything seems to be about timing – from the early stages, when you chart the days since your last period and try to make love at the 'right' moment, to the countdown to your first IVF treatment. For many women who are starting the process in their late thirties or early forties, time is of the essence in a very real way. Indeed, it's the feeling of 'time running out', and the consequent pressure this causes that often brings them to my practice. Julia Bueno, a psychotherapist, sees this with her clients, too, and acknowledges the intense focus on the body that initiating treatment entails.

She says: 'When fertility can't be taken for granted, the process of conception becomes one that women have to think about in greater detail. It often has to be taken in stages, so women begin to focus on their hormones, whether they are producing the right number of follicles, the right amount of womb lining, and so on. This makes it almost impossible not to respond emotionally to each stage of fertility treatment.'

In order to regain a sense of control over what's happening to you (while still accepting that the ultimate result is out of your control – a tricky balance to strike), constructing a time line will make a huge difference to the way you view your treatment.

When I first say the words 'time line' to my clients, it can put them in mind of a science-fiction novel or make them think of work. But it can be one of the most effective stress-relieving tools you can use, especially if you are about to start treatment such as IVF, IUI (intrauterine insemination), Clomid, or any of the other processes with a defined time scale and build-up. It is also an intensely practical way of putting yourself in the best possible physical and mental state, and works especially well with those who like structure and to feel that they're 'doing something'.

How to create your own time line

- Draw a long line on a large piece of paper (or across two pages of your journal).
- At the start, write today's date. At the far end of the line, write the date you consider to be the end of this particular treatment cycle. If you're going through IVF, for example, this could be day 15 or 16 after embryo transfer.
- Along the line, write down the dates of the medical part of your treatment, e.g. 'start nasal spray', or 'scan'.
- Once you've inserted all the practical information, ask yourself, 'How will I make sure that I am doing something positive on every single one of those days along the line? What do I want the next six weeks to look like – physically, mentally, emotionally and spiritually?'
- Brainstorm a list of activities and resources on a separate piece of paper. It could include things like 'have a massage', 'go for coffee with neighbour', 'attend a fertility support group', 'call mum', etc.
- Now insert these activities into your time line, thinking about what you might need most, and when. So, say you're having your embryo transfer on a particular date, you may want to have your activity as 'one hour visualisation to music' or 'call friend from support group', rather than 'go for a swim' or "go to the pub'.

Sample time line

No two patients are exactly alike and, therefore, no two patient treatment plans will be the same. Below is a standard IVF cycle outline that summarises the important steps involved in treatment.

1. **Birth control pills** (approx. 14-21 days).

2. **Synarel/Lupron** (approx. 12–15 days).
Drugs used to 'shut down' the menstrual cycle, may cause symptoms akin to menopause e.g. hot flushes and headache

3) **Baseline ultrasound**

4. **Stimulation** (approx. 10–12 days).
Ovaries stimulated and monitored via daily injections, may cause symptoms akin to premenstrual syndrom

5) **Trigger shot**

6. **Egg retrieval** (36–37 hours after trigger shot).
Usually done under general anaesthetic

7. **Embryo transfer** (3-5 days after retrieval).
Relatively simple procedure, clinics may recommend rest afterwards up to a few days. Start off using Progesterone either pessary or injection form.

8. **Pregnancy test** (14 days after retrieval).

9) **Ultrasounds**
1st: approx. 6 1/2–7 weeks pregnant
2nd: approx. 7 1/2–8 1/2 weeks pregnant.
Release to OB at 8-10 weeks pregnant.

An IVF cycle will vary hugely from person to person and should be seen as a series of procedures and 'hurdles' rather than as a one-off event. Monitoring of the individual will mean that time frames may well change between each of these stages and a great degree of flexibility around other commitments is to be strongly recommended. At certain stages a person may well be in the clinic at least once a day. An IVF cycle is incredibly time consuming.

Remember: these dates will need to be flexible during treatment, as dates are nearly always a rough guide only.

One of my clients was a practising Muslim and she found drawing up a time line useful in terms of her spiritual support. By planning the build-up to treatment before the month of Ramadan, she was able to plot the physical and social activities she'd identified as helpful to her, and was in a positive and spiritual place when egg transfer finally happened.

Please bear in mind that putting something on your time line every day doesn't mean filling it with frantic activity. What matters is that it's your choice how you spend that time, and by planning it in advance, even if you decide to do nothing, you have more of a sense of control than if you left it to chance. The treatment process puts you in a relatively powerless situation as it is (and for many of you, this may be the first time you've had so little control over your life). By approaching your days mindfully and strategically, you've pulled back a bit of power, which is important for many women and men struggling to conceive.

The time line is also a great place to apply the 80/20 rule. One of the questions I'm most frequently asked in my support groups is: 'What should I be doing in order to give myself the best possible chance of success?' Of course, the answer to that will be different for everyone, and it's true that putting the best-quality foods and supplements in your mouth, and the most nourishing and positive thoughts in your head, will maximise your chances. But don't go overboard. So, yes, for 80% of your time, it's great to put exercise into your time line and to eat organic food and meditate and do affirmations. But you're only human, and striving to get it 'right' will only create anxiety and tension, which will ultimately work against you. So make sure you add trips to the pub, or to the cake shop, or whatever your particular pleasure is, and allow yourself a grumble on the phone to a friend. Indulged in sparingly, these activities will actually make you feel better the rest of the time and help you to connect with the outside world.

Your support team

A top athlete would never dream of entering a race without thorough preparation. They would make sure they were in top physical and mental condition, whatever their discipline, and to do this they would need a team of people around them to ensure they were in the best possible shape. This would include trainers, physiotherapists, sports coaches, masseurs, nutritionists – and, of course, family and friends cheering from the sidelines.

Your race may not be of Olympic proportions (at least, not physically) but it is nonetheless important that you have a support team to help you, and who will be on your side regardless of what happens in the final battle.

Your team will probably be made up of clinical professionals, friends, family – and possibly alternative therapists. But only you can decide. I like to visualise my support team in terms of a circle with concentric bands running through it. So, right at the centre, I have my partner and my fertility consultant at the clinic. Then, in the next ring, I have good friends, close family and a woman I met on an online forum who has become an invaluable source of support. In the next is my acupuncturist, other friends, helpline nurses, etc.

If you're having difficulty working out who should be on your support team, it may help to think back to the last time you dealt with a really tough situation. You may not have gone through anything like fertility treatment before, but most people have suffered at least one of the more unpleasant but commonplace life events, such as losing a family member, going through a relationship break-up or experiencing financial difficulties. Who was by your side at that time? Or, if your circle of friends has changed since then, who do you feel would be good in a crisis now? I am fortunate to have a number of wonderful friends in my life, but I wouldn't have included them all in my support team. Some, for example, mean well but can't stop themselves from giving advice; others are fabulous company on a night out but aren't the first people I'd turn to when I was feeling low.

Another thing to bear in mind is the level of support you feel comfortable with. For some people, support means a daily phone conversation; for others, it is meeting up for coffee once a month. For others still, support is a more intangible concept – it can be information. I even put 'statistics' as part of my support team, as the fact that so many other people were going through what I was, and that I wasn't an abnormal freak, was comforting to remember.

Using your support team

Once you've identified who you want on your team, you need to think about how they're going to support you. One of my clients chose three people from her close 'circles' and decided to phone one (her mother) and text the other two after every appointment at the clinic. For some of you, that might be way too much. I probably fell somewhere in the middle in my support needs. Because I'd made a note of who was on my team, I was able to incorporate seeing or phoning them into my time line, helping me feel supported and encouraged on a regular basis. When I went for egg collection, I visualised all my support team cheering me on and willing the treatment to succeed. It certainly helped me through what most people acknowledge can be a traumatic process.

Julia Bueno, the psychotherapist we met earlier in this chapter, is a strong believer in the power of the support team: 'Ultimately, I think if a woman notes what and how she is feeling in the process, and keeps talking to supportive people and drawing as much nourishment as possible from all around her, this will help to keep her afloat at what can be an unbearably stressful time,' she says.

Here are some of her tips for holding it together:

- Keep up the things that make you feel happy and grounded, so fertility treatments and issues don't overwhelm you: seeing friends, exercise, work, and so on.
- Talk to others who have gone/are going through their own fertility struggles – either in person or on fertility sites. You aren't alone.
- However hellish a treatment may feel, remember that each stage of it is, potentially, 'progress'. I used to say this to myself when injecting every day – if I weren't doing this, I'd have no chance of becoming pregnant.
- Limit the amount you read about fertility. Information overload can add to stress rather than relieve it, and you may end up living in a bubble for fear of limiting your chances of conceiving. I believe that the odd glass of wine may actually provide useful stress relief for some.

CASE STUDY

Angela is a former client of mine who is still undergoing treatment and yet has managed to take her thinking (and even her body) into a more positive and resourceful place through doing these exercises and really engaging with the process.

ANGELA'S STORY

When I started fertility treatment at the age of 45, I had recently married my husband and knew I wanted a baby more than anything, so I was devastated to discover that because of my age, I wouldn't be allowed to use my own eggs. I had no idea that this was UK protocol, and none of the NHS consultants or GPs informed me of this until it was too late. We really didn't know anything at this stage, certainly none of the technical terms such as AMH [anti-*müllerian* hormone] or LH [luteinizing hormone], or what the treatment really involved. We ended up going to a private clinic where the consultant said they'd consider IUI rather than IVF.

My husband is from Zimbabwe and is a very private person – he's not used to talking about his feelings, so it's been quite a challenge for him. But he listened to Anya when I don't think I could have convinced him, so having an independent third party has definitely helped. He's also made changes in the way he communicates with his family as a result. He was so embarrassed when she asked how often we had sex, and I said: 'Well, we're newly-weds, so we're at it like rabbits!' But it was good to hear we were doing the right thing – apparently, one of the reasons people struggle to conceive is that they only have sex between days 10 and 14.

Going through this process has been a rollercoaster of emotions. One thing that helped was to identify the strengths I'd developed in hard times in the past. It was good to acknowledge that I am a strong, determined and focused person and I need to draw on all of that for the journey ahead. For example, I'd lost 14 stone and in doing so cured myself of polycystic ovary syndrome; I'd survived losing my mother, my business failing, a divorce, major surgery and doing a degree, all in a short space of time. Just knowing I'd got through all of that and emerged a stronger person has given me more confidence in my own resilience.

I've also learnt to challenge the experts – at first I felt guilty, as you think they know everything and you shouldn't question them, but I now feel I can ask things, and I actually managed to bring forward a treatment cycle just by not taking no for an answer.

I've had lots of alternative therapies – reiki, reflexology, NLP [neuro-linguistic programming] – and I've also been to see a nutritionist and a healer. It's taught me to look after myself. I'm a 'wired and tired' type of person – I just go like the clappers and then collapse – but that's no way to get pregnant. So I've learnt things that are good for me generally, as well as making it more likely that I'll conceive. It was also important for me to know I could say 'It wasn't meant to be' if our treatment is ultimately unsuccessful. A year from now, I will know that I've tried everything in my power – without being neurotic. I won't be looking back and saying, 'If only I'd read that book or done that course'.

I know I delayed having a baby because I didn't want to repeat the mistakes my own mother made; mine was not a happy childhood. But I've done a lot of work around that and my fears have totally changed. I now know I will be a brilliant mum, whether it happens through fertility treatment or some other way.

Internal or external processing?

If there's one thing I want you to take from this book, it's that fertility treatment is an individual and personal journey, and that we all adapt to it in different ways. These days, it can feel almost compulsory to tell everyone you meet about any difficulties you're experiencing. But we all process information and emotions differently, and people tend to split broadly into two types – internal and external.

It's not difficult to work out which camp you fall into. When you have a problem, do you tend to mull it over first, telling people after the event, or do you need to share your thoughts and anxieties in order to find a solution? I tend towards the latter – if I'm unhappy about something, most of my close friends and family know about it and I look to them for ideas and advice. But that's just me, and if you prefer to deal with things yourself first, it doesn't make you wrong. To make a sweeping generalisation, women tend to be more external processors while men keep things bottled up more and deal with their feelings in different ways, such as physical activity or talking to other men about unrelated subjects (such as football). Of course, there are also many women who process internally and men externally. But the point is it doesn't matter *how* you do it – so long as you feel happy with the amount and quality of support you are getting. So, the time line of an internally focused person might consist of activities such as going for long walks or reading books on nutrition and relaxation, whereas their externally focused counterpart may prefer to attend support groups or call helplines. There's no right or wrong – just choose what feels like a comfortable level of support for you.

Powerchange tool: riches inventory

The riches inventory is a fantastic way to gain a greater awareness of your resources, both past and present, and helps you to view your situation in a more positive and thankful way. Yes, it is possible!

Under the headings below, write a few words or sentences that exemplify the insights and gifts you have gained in each area. Try to find something positive or constructive even from a bad experience. For example, you might have had a difficult childhood and felt abandoned by your parents. But maybe that has instilled in you a sense of resilience and independence you can draw on in your current situation? Or, conversely, maybe you were an indulged only child, which has left you with a strong sense of security and the idea you were valuable and loved? You may be surprised to find just how resourceful you really are.

Past resources inventory

Upbringing:..

Social background:..

Religion:...

Nationality/cultural resources:..

Other:...

....

Key experiences and learning

Travel:...

....

....

Three significant people:...

....

....

Three traumatic/painful experiences:.......................................

....

....

Three really happy experiences:...

....

....

Three unusual experiences:...

....

....

Present resources inventory

Material possessions: ....

Three abilities: ....

Friends and colleagues: ....

Three skills:..

Attitudes: ....

New/recent insights into resources you are just realising you have:

....

....

Expected future resources inventory

Opportunities: ....

Time: ....

Other:..

Resource development

What one resource would you particularly like to develop?

....

Action? ....

What single resource has been significantly neglected or forgotten?

....

Action? ....

....

What needs to happen for these hidden resources to become practical and active for you?

....

....

....

CHAPTER 6

KEEP IT TOGETHER: RESPECT YOUR RELATIONSHIP

"A loving heart is the truest wisdom."
Charles Dickens

When you and your partner decided to try for a baby together, you probably didn't imagine you'd end up where you are now (unless, of course, you were always aware of a medical problem that would prevent you from conceiving naturally). For most couples, the biggest decision is, 'When shall we stop using contraception?' rather than, 'How long before we consider donation or adoption?' Even the strongest relationships can be rocked by one of you feeling low, depressed or anxious – and now there are two of you experiencing extreme and often conflicting emotions. Sadly, some relationships do fall apart, but it is possible to remain together, and even strengthen your bond, if you are aware of some of the possible pitfalls, and make the time and effort to see things from your partner's perspective.

Some warning signs to look out for include:

■ Over-reliance on your partner – expecting them to be everything to you.
■ Under-reliance – completely avoiding talking about the situation.
■ Losing perspective of yourselves as a couple outside of your fertility issues.
■ Losing sight of what attracted you to your partner in the early days.
■ Thinking of your partner, rather than the infertility, as the problem.

When my husband, Damion, and I were confronted with our first diagnosis of infertility, it appeared that the problem lay solely with him. An operation on a torsion he had had as a teenager had apparently left him with no viable sperm and he was totally devastated when he found out. Having children had always been part of our plan and it never occurred to either of us that it wouldn't be possible. Damion fell apart and blamed himself, saying that he felt totally emasculated and that I should go and find someone else to have children with.

It was heartbreaking to see him in this state (and I know of many other couples where the husband has reacted in a similar manner). I knew I couldn't fix the situation or make it better for him: all I could do was to reassure him that it was our problem and that we were going to get through it together. It may be tempting to point fingers and assign blame (particularly if one person in the relationship has left it 'too late' or has made choices they feel may have damaged their ability to reproduce), but it only leads to deeper damage in the long term. Of course, you may well be feeling angry (it can help to express this anger in your journal, or to a counsellor, coach or trusted friend), and if you are, it's important to acknowledge it. But getting stuck in blame makes it much harder to work together as a team, something that's essential if you want to come out of this process with your relationship intact.

In the previous chapter, we looked at external and internal processing, and relationships are a key area in which the way you handle your communication can be almost as important as the meaning of your words. It's the done thing in this day and age to resolve a situation by 'talking it through' – but for many people, this is actually counterproductive. Forcing someone who doesn't want to talk to 'open up' can actually make them withdraw further and possibly promote the kind of behaviour you were struggling with in the first place. Knowing whether or not your partner is a 'talker' – and respecting them as they are - can be a wonderful gift to any relationship, let alone one in which you are both experiencing feelings that cut to the heart of your identity and sense of self.

Patricia Love and Steven Stosny have written a great book, *Why Women Talk and Men Walk*,[1] about communication differences between the sexes, and I highly recommend it for couples who are struggling to get 'on the same wavelength' but don't want to spend hours in circular discussions that go nowhere.

It's also important to acknowledge your partner as a separate being, with their own feelings, thoughts and needs. This can be a huge strain for some people, especially at a time when you feel needier than ever. And, of course, this may be exacerbated by the medication you are taking at various stages of your treatment. The truth is, you may not be able to give your partner everything they need – and they may not be able to satisfy your needs completely, either.

For some couples, this is the first time they have encountered such a conflict, and the only counsel I can give here is to be gentle with yourself and your partner. You are perfectly within your rights to have expectations of another person, and to ask for what you want and need. But you must also be prepared for the possibility that it is not in their power at that particular time to meet your needs, and you will have to look to yourself or a friend or family member to do that. I realise that this flies in the face of the popular belief that love conquers all and that well-matched couples never need anyone outside their relationship. But my experience tells me that even the happiest of relationships go through periods of conflict and strain, and giving yourself a hard time when you and your partner can't be everything to each other only makes things worse. By asking yourself, 'What do I need right now and who can give it to me?' you are taking a step towards greater responsibility for your own emotional wellbeing – and, often, taking the pressure off your partner leads to them feeling freer and more able to meet your needs in the end.

Exercise

Assess your own expectations and relationship patterns by jotting down in your journal the answers to the following questions:

- What do you need right now (both physically and emotionally)?
- What do you think your partner is able to give you?
- If there is a discrepancy between these two answers, who else can you ask to meet that need? (I am thinking about a close friend, coach or an organisation – not suggesting you have an affair!)
- Think of an occasion in the past when you have had conflicting needs or desires. What happened? How did you resolve the tension?
- How could you apply that knowledge to your current situation?
- If you haven't experienced anything similar in the past, imagine what course of action you might suggest to your best friend if they were in your situation.

Treatment-specific conflicts

IVF and other types of fertility treatment are among the greatest scientific advances in recent decades, to my mind at least, but they also bring their own conflicts and challenges. Our value systems (and often those of our parents, strangely enough) can come into question when we are faced with difficult decisions about reproduction. To what lengths would we be willing to go to have a child? Would we consider IUI but not IVF? Sperm but not an egg donor? Adoption but not a surrogate? Each of these options involves moral and ethical issues that we may never have considered before, and our thinking can change and develop over the course of several months.

These treatment options can be highly emotive and we react to them from the gut. We often say something 'sits right' with us – or not – without necessarily being able to explain why. This is why it is so important (and often so difficult) to respect the responses of your partner. Not only do you come to the relationship with your own values, expectations, moral and cultural upbringing and education, but they do, too. When you come to think of it, it's actually quite unlikely that you will happen to agree with your partner on every single issue. Cast your mind back to the thought processes that led you to where you are now, and appreciate that it may take the same amount of time, or longer, for your partner to catch up. Be prepared, too, for the possibility that they will never share your view on certain issues. But give them time – as I said before, feelings change.

Angela, who we met in Chapter 5, saw her husband perform a complete u-turn on the idea of using a donor egg if they needed it, to the extent that he has promised that if they do succeed in having a baby, he will donate sperm for other couples experiencing fertility problems. And this comes from a man whose cultural background was absolutely against such 'intervention'. I'm not saying that your partner will necessarily come to see everything from your perspective, but by giving them the gift of time and the opportunity to research the options *in a way that is meaningful to them*, you stand a better chance of seeing eye-to-eye. Think about it – when do you feel most open to new ideas? When you have the space and freedom to think things through for yourself, or when you feel your opinions are not respected and you are being browbeaten into changing them?

It can also help to try to practise what may initially feel like the impossible, and listen to the emotion behind what your partner is saying, rather than taking the words as gospel. Just before Damion and I set off for egg retrieval, he went into an emotional tailspin, telling me repeatedly, 'I can't do it'. Of course, at the time, his words upset me, but looking back, we both realise that he was utterly overwhelmed and felt powerless over the experience, and that he didn't literally mean, 'I don't want to go through with the treatment'. He needed acknowledgement that he was also going through a major trauma, and what came out at that moment was a lot of pent-up anxiety and frustration.

The one thing I'd like you to take from this chapter is that conflict and emotional swings are quite normal. What would be less normal, in fact, would be if you both breezed through fertility treatment without a care in the world. I'm not saying you should go looking for trouble, but try to be kind to yourself and your partner when difficulties do arise.

Exercise: magic-mirror triangle

This is a powerful exercise that enables you to see an issue from someone else's point of view – quite literally. Because it works on a kinaesthetic level, it can give you profound insight and it accesses the unconscious mind in an astounding way. You can use it for any issue and for any other person. Do the exercise alone, or with someone else reading out the prompts, but make sure the person with you isn't the one you are having the issue with, or things could get a little complicated. You need to be somewhere you feel safe, able to let go and experience what comes up. Give it as much time as it needs.

- Choose a spot in the room where you have plenty of space around you. This is where 'you' will stay – let's call it position 1.
- Imagine the person you want to understand better standing directly in front of you, about two metres away. For the sake of this exercise, we will assume this is your partner, but you can do it for relationships with your parents, friends, or even abstract concepts such as money or sex. Your partner is standing in position 2.

■ From position 1, look across and visualise your partner standing opposite you. What do you notice when you look at them? What do you feel? What do you want to say to them? You can say it aloud or write it down. Spend a few minutes absorbing everything you think and feel about this person right now.

■ Step off position 1 and stamp around in a circle. Shake out all the feelings.

■ Walk over to where you imagine your partner to be, in position 2. You are now them, looking back at you. What do you, as your partner, notice about the you standing in position 1? What do you feel? What do you think about that person? What do you want to say to them? Again, spend a few moments just being your partner; say what you feel aloud or write it down.

■ Step off position 2, stamp around and shake out those feelings.

■ Stand in a spot about two metres away from positions 1 and 2, making the point of a triangle. This is position 3. You are neither you nor your partner, but a neutral observer.

■ What do you want to say? Looking at you and your partner from a distance, and having heard what you both think and feel, what do you notice? What does the you in position 1 need to know? Again, say it out loud or write it down. Make sure you tell them everything – however long it takes.

■ It can be useful to create an anchor to help you absorb this knowledge. Once you've said all you need to say and you feel at peace with it, press the thumb and forefinger of your right hand together, as you, all-knowing, all-understanding, look over at yourself in position 1.

■ Walk back again to position 1 and integrate the new knowledge you have absorbed into your mind and body. Touch your thumb and forefinger together to make the feeling stronger and seal it into your consciousness. Look over at your partner in position 2. What do you want to say to them now?

■ Walk over to position 2 and look back at yourself in position 1. What do you see, think, feel?

You can go between positions 1 and 2 as often as feels right, or repeat the entire exercise. The first time you try this, it can feel very powerful, but you will benefit from its repetition and go even deeper into your emotions, bringing up and resolving issues you weren't previously aware of.

IVF and the single person

I must confess that I'm no expert on dealing with IVF as a single person, and I have nothing but admiration for those who are prepared to take on the process without a partner. To some extent, the stakes are higher than for couples – both financially and emotionally – but there are also positives to undertaking fertility treatment alone. For example, there is less potential for conflict, as you will make all the decisions concerning your treatment and parenting, which can be a cause of stress in a partnership. For many women, it is the most empowering thing they have done in their lives, and it makes them feel more complete to know they are not compromising by finding a partner merely to act as a sperm donor.

I have several friends who are approaching their mid- to late-thirties who have chosen to freeze their eggs so they have the choice to 'go it alone' if they are still single in a few years. But just because you will be making all the decisions doesn't mean you won't need people to be there for you, and it's crucial to identify your support team (see Chapter 5) as early as possible.

Choose your team wisely – pick people who will make you feel confident in your decision and won't offer moral judgements. You may also want to join specific threads on Internet forums for single people undergoing fertility treatment. There are many others out there following the same path, and the support and encouragement of those who have gone before can be enormously helpful.

Exercise: honour the mentor

It can be tempting in times of stress to look outside ourselves for reassurance and solutions, forgetting that we are actually wise beings. This exercise is designed to bring out the wise elder in you, and give you confidence in your own thinking. It can be wonderful to make decisions based on this intuitive wisdom, as it will feel right and make sense in a way that external advice, with its conflicts and confusion, might not. As I've said before – trust yourself.
Find a place to relax, maybe sitting in bed or in a comfortable chair. Have your journal and a pen to hand. Close your eyes.

- Imagine a video of your life. To help you get into it, try to visualise what has happened so far today. Watch it on the screen behind your eyelids, and try to remember the details.
- Now fast-forward that video to 10 years down the line. What do you look like? What are your surroundings like? What are you doing?
- Have the future you address the camera directly – he/she is looking right at you. What do you want to ask him/her? What is his/her response? What does he/she think about the situation you're in right now?
- Open your eyes and write what the older you had to say in your journal.

I often repeat this exercise for other issues in my life, but when I was going through IVF, I remember writing down: 'Everything is normal; there will be an end; you're stronger than you think you are. Go gently with Damion: he's doing his best.' It felt calming and reassuring, and it gave me a sense of peace no amount of reading could.

As every couple is different, it's hard to provide general solutions, but it might be worth bearing in mind some of the following when considering your relationship:

1. Try not to expect too much from each other: you are going through this experience both as individuals and as a couple.
2. Keep short, honest and open accounts with each other; don't let resentment build up.
3. Focus on the aspects of the other person that you love, and make a point of having fun together.
4. Get as much outside help as you need, whether it's a counsellor, coach or other third party.
5. Try to visit the clinic together as much as possible – there is still a tendency to sideline men in the treatment process, and being there for each other can be tremendously affirming.

CHAPTER 7

MAN TO MAN: THE MALE PERSPECTIVE

"A successful man is one who can lay a firm foundation with the bricks others have thrown at him."
David Brinkley (American journalist)

This chapter is all about men and for men, about their responses to the diagnosis of infertility and how best they can be helped. It features personal accounts from several men who share their experiences of struggling to conceive, either with their own fertility problems or as the partner of a woman receiving treatment. As some of this chapter is obviously written by a woman, I hope the case studies you read here will speak to you more eloquently and helpfully than I could ever hope to.

We know that men and women are different – but these differences often become more polarised when a couple are having trouble conceiving. Under stress, we all tend to cope in more 'gendered' ways – women reach out as men become more distant – so it is hardly surprising that fertility treatment highlights the gender divide so starkly.

Pip Reilly, a counsellor at the Bridge Centre in London with years of experience working with both couples and individuals undergoing fertility treatment, is convinced that the only way to bridge the gulf between the sexes is to understand and respect each other's differences. 'The male has masculinity and ego and the female needs to understand her emotion,' he says. 'The two opposites, at best, complement each other. At worst, a wedge goes between the two. I would say something like 50% of the couples I've seen have ended up on the rocks because of fertility issues, and that is particularly down to inability to communicate.'

Pip has found that during the first IVF cycle, partners tend to rely on each other for support. When it comes to the second cycle, the statistics remain largely the same. By the time they reach the third cycle, the majority of women have turned to friends as their primary support, while the men continue to look to their female partners to help them cope. Tired of 'coping for two', the women forge more diverse external links where their emotional needs can be better met; the men, whether from shame, fear or a combination of the two, close ranks and tend to isolate themselves.

Sammy Lee, in his book *Counselling in Male Infertility*[2] (which we will hear from in more detail later in the chapter), notes: 'Men are generally reluctant to consider support, let alone formal support such as counselling. [They] seem to want to cope on their own, resenting intrusion.' At the time of writing, in 1996, Sammy found that men were more receptive to more distanced, one-way communication such as newsletters. These days, the first place people tend to go for information is the Internet, which has the added bonus of enabling men to communicate with another person while retaining a physical and psychological distance.

Pip Reilly founded Mensfe,[3] a website that gives men dealing with infertility a place to find the information they're looking for and the opportunity to ask questions and share stories on the forums and blogs. However, for many men, simply reading others' personal accounts is challenging enough. Pip says:

> I noticed one blogger wrote something on the boards bemoaning the fact that there were very few new conversations and yet he knew there were more and more men reading the blogs as the site numbers had increased. One guy came back to him and said, 'You have the capacity to tell your story and articulate it very well. It's not that we are not there with you, it's just that we can't do it.' And that was an incredible statement. It is simply very difficult for a man to communicate on this level.

The topics on Mensfe's forums range from 'women's reactions to male infertility' to 'dealing with doctors' and even 'funny stories', further evidence (as we saw in Chapter 1) that humour can be a real lifeline when you're struggling with issues that strike at your very core. The tone of the posts is friendly and supportive, but you certainly wouldn't mistake it for a women's chat room. Other than the 'general discussion' topic, the largest numbers of posts are found in the 'funny' or 'let off some steam' sections, which may be indicative of the need for men to find emotional release anonymously where they feel it would be inappropriate or simply impossible with their partners.

The supportive male partner

While there may be similarities in the ways in which men typically react to the news that conceiving might not be as straightforward as they had hoped, there is a huge difference between discovering it's your partner who has the issue and being told that the 'fault' lies with you.

Men whose sperm test results are satisfactory may experience an initial sense of relief, as they do not feel their masculinity has been affected in the way it can be when there are problems with their sperm. However, this relief is often followed by feelings of powerlessness and fear that they are unable to support their partner as they would wish.

In group-therapy sessions, Pip reports that men are:

> terrified of saying the wrong thing. Hormones are running high, emotions are running high, and one of the major things they share is their fear of not knowing how to help their partner. They may think, 'Okay, I'll give them a cuddle.' And the cuddle's wrong. They may sit down over dinner and try to connect – but it's an inopportune time to talk. So the analogy they use is that it's like walking on a razor's edge and they could fall off either side at any time'.

CASE STUDY

Let's hear from Will, who found himself cast in the role of 'strong supporter' while he and his wife were going through treatment.

WILL'S STORY

The greatest problem at the beginning was that they never found a specific reason why we couldn't get pregnant. My sperm test was fine, and although my wife had a reduced ovarian store, it wasn't impossible it could happen naturally. But because we'd been trying for a year, and the view was that if we were going to have IVF it would be better sooner rather than later, we went ahead quite early, relative to other couples. There was also a lot of pressure and anxiety about wanting to get pregnant and it not happening, so we were keen to do something proactive. I think the chances of us conceiving naturally were probably reduced because there was so much tension around.

I realise things were different for me, because I hadn't been thinking about having a child for years and years, whereas my wife had. She was more pessimistic about it possibly not happening, maybe because she'd thought about it a lot. I was just hoping she'd get pregnant, so I didn't really pay attention to the details, such as how long we'd been trying. But we were both keen to get on with what would give us the best chance (in our case, IVF), and that was what the clinic recommended. We didn't want to try other treatments if we would eventually end up having IVF anyway. I'm glad we took that approach and began treatment when we did – trying to conceive naturally had become quite depressing.

I didn't really talk to anyone other than my wife about it in any great depth. I mentioned it to a couple of friends, but not the minutiae. I had to talk to people at work about it as I would need to take time off, but it wouldn't have been my mindset to discuss it with loads of people anyway.

My experience of the clinic was essentially fine, but I imagine it's very different if there is an identifiable problem with the male partner. When there's nothing wrong with your sperm, there's only so much you can do – you just end up supporting your partner. They did offer us counselling but at that stage neither of us felt we wanted it. Maybe if things had gone on longer, we might have said yes. But I know my wife got a lot of support from INUK [Infertility Network UK].

Before each treatment cycle, I would stop drinking, take lots of zinc tablets and eat a healthy diet, which got a bit depressing as it went on for such a long time. Mentally, I certainly felt that it was necessary to build up towards the possibility that it might not work, which I guess was important for me but also so I could support my wife if things didn't go well. There were definitely times when I felt that I needed to be strong enough to look after both of us.

The process you have to go through in order to get the necessary bits together in the test tube is very odd. They did the sperm tests and then there were two more occasions when I had to provide a sample for the treatment, and it definitely became more stressful then. You get shown into this slightly grubby room with second-hand porn mags lying around – it's definitely not fun. But I acknowledge it's a relatively minor part of the stresses involved in the whole process.

We went through three cycles, one with a frozen embryo, and we'd decided we'd do one more after that. If it didn't work, that would be it. We had talked about adoption, but as we went along it became more difficult to imagine, as we were so focused on the process of having our own child. But I'm absolutely sure we'd have done it in the end. As it is, the cycle with the frozen embryo was successful and we now have a beautiful baby daughter.

In retrospect, I think it would have been more helpful for my wife had I engaged more in the details of the treatment. It was probably part of my coping mechanism – if I didn't know much about it, I didn't have to worry about it, but of course it meant she was unfairly burdened with the knowledge. Then again, maybe that distance helped me support her better.

I honestly don't think that fertility treatment can ever be a pleasant experience. The most important thing, whatever the outcome, is to try to recognise that there is life beyond IVF.

The infertile male

The adjective that crops up time and time again when describing the man who has either no sperm, or poor-quality sperm that hinder conception, is 'isolated'. According to Sammy Lee:

Men's right to be supreme is challenged in cases of male infertility, so not only is the diagnosis a shock, his male ideology as a whole is also challenged. Thus the whole idea of being a man is at stake – effectively, a man's entire self-belief system is demolished with one blow, thereby placing him in a state of crisis.

This 'crisis' will typically manifest itself in depression, anger and, sometimes, impotence. Sammy estimates that up to 25% of couples experience problems with sex when the male partner's infertility is identified. Feeling less of a man, and with the 'reason' for intercourse gone, he may see his libido plummet, causing further anxiety within the relationship. He may also be affected by his friends trying to trivialise or make a joke of his feelings (a common response is for them to offer to 'help out with the wife'). It is small wonder, therefore, that Sammy identifies siblings as being a good source of emotional support for the infertile man – parents may well be too wrapped up in their desire for grandchildren to see the matter clearly, while sensitive male friends are, sadly, rare.

CASE STUDY

My husband, Damion, was lucky in that he did have good male friends to talk to and, perhaps unusually, was willing to open up to a counsellor. Here's his story.

DAMION'S STORY

I first knew there was some kind of problem when we'd been trying for a while and I went to my GP for a check-up. He was pretty blunt when he delivered the results – basically, he said there was no sperm in the sample they'd tested. He obviously had no idea how to handle it and was really brutal. I felt like I'd been kicked in the gut, it was such a blow.

I'd thought there might be a problem as I'd had an operation on a torsion, where the tubes in the testicles are twisted, when I was 16. They'd said it might cause problems in later life, but I didn't really take any notice at the time. I'm glad I didn't, now, as that would have really affected my relationships and how I viewed myself – it would have limited me in lots of ways.

From the moment of diagnosis, Anya and I went off at different angles. She was very action-based and immediately started looking into options, whereas I was still very emotional. So, at her suggestion, we went to see a specialist who did a biopsy on me. I was told that what had happened when I was 16 was almost like I'd had a vasectomy. But the specialist was hopeful, as they did find some live sperm they could work with.

I remember I was an emotional wreck - my identity was very much tied up with being able to have children. Looking back, I let it define me, and I wish I'd understood at the time that your identity isn't dependent on your circumstances.

I knew how desperately Anya wanted children and I became a bit of a martyr, saying: 'We should call it a day. You should go off and have kids with someone else.' I'd get cards from friends announcing births or they'd tell me about pregnancies, and I'd think: 'You lucky sods.' I know you shouldn't begrudge people, but I did - all I wanted was for us to have children and it was difficult to climb out of that situation.

At the time, we didn't know anyone else who was going through the same thing. I did manage to find a male counsellor who was very supportive, and my friends were really good, but I deliberately talked about different things when I was out with them. They helped remind me who I was, rather than just a body with hardly any sperm, but I would have appreciated the chance to talk to other men in my situation.

It was important for me to actually do things to make myself feel better, and to focus on our relationship, which is why I'm glad I didn't know about the problem before we were married. It's crucial to do normal stuff like go out for a drink or see a band - not to

> pretend 'Everything's normal, everything's fine,' but to remember who you are, other than one half of an infertile couple.
>
> In retrospect, I think it would have helped to look at ways I'd got through difficult situations in the past, as I know that was useful for Anya. And I'd say to any women reading this that men need to be reassured that the relationship is about more than having children. We love to hear how good we are at things and how much we mean to you. I needed to hear that our relationship was more important and that we could deal with this together.

I asked Damion if he could think of any advice or coping strategies to offer to male readers. Here are his tips for getting through:

- Infertility is a medical condition. It is not your fault. Please write this down and remember it when things are tough. You may feel guilty, but *it's not your fault*.
- Try to remember that your partner is with you because she wants to be, and because of the man you are. She fell in love with you before you started thinking about children and that love is not contingent upon whether or not you can have any.
- Don't punish yourself. Try to redefine yourself by your interests, your beliefs, you friends and family. Learn to enjoy being you and give yourself a break.
- You are allowed to feel the way you do. If things are too painful for you to discuss with your partner, try to find a counsellor or therapist. Talking to a stranger with an objective viewpoint and no agenda can be immensely liberating.
- Decide for yourself what you can and cannot deal with emotionally in terms of treatment options. Be realistic and honest, whatever you think your partner would like to hear, and don't let anyone pressure you. Some of these decisions will affect the rest of your life – and potentially the lives of others.

■ Keep yourself fit and healthy to optimise your chances of conceiving. You'll probably feel better and look better, too, which can be important at a time when the ego is taking a battering.

Donor insemination

Donor insemination (DI) is used for a variety of male infertility issues, including when a man has no sperm and it is unlikely that surgery to retrieve any would be successful (irreversible azoospermia). In terms of fertility treatment, it is often considered a last resort and, for some, a step too far on the road to conceiving your own biological child. It also has significant repercussions, both physically and psychologically, so everyone who chooses DI must undertake mandatory counselling. So many questions arise with this option – both for the woman (will my partner leave me and the child if it's not biologically his? Will he consider the donor a rival? How will this affect our wider family and friends: will they understand? Will I still feel the same about my partner?) and the man (will I love this child enough? Will we feel like a proper family? What will my friends/family/colleagues think? How will our child react if/when we tell them?).

Sammy Lee has counselled many men going through DI, and says that although a few come easily to a decision, the majority agonise over it for some time. In his experience, it is most often the female partner who initiates DI treatment, and he claims, 'The vast majority of men have grave reservations about DI, although they may agree to accept the treatment' viewing it as a kind of 'gift'.

Couples (or, indeed, single people) in the UK looking for information and support about donor conception will find case studies and material on the Donor Conception Network (DCN) website,[4] which also includes information for single women and a section dedicated to men.

CASE STUDY

Lee (not to be confused with Sammy Lee) reached out to the DCN when he was confronting the implications of fathering a child with donated sperm.

LEE'S STORY

I'd had a nagging doubt at the back of my mind about my fertility, particularly since Kate and I had been trying for a baby for what seemed like years and nothing was happening. It came as a shock when I was diagnosed as having azoospermia (no sperm in the ejaculate) in August 2007. Both my wife and I were totally shell-shocked and shed many tears as we realised that we were pretty much no longer in control of the whole family-planning thing.

I was born with undescended testes and then had a torsion when I was 14 that required corrective surgery. After many months of trying without success, I decided to look at the internet for information about torsions. I was shocked to read something about 'compromised fertility'. Nobody had ever said anything about that to me. Because of my history, I had a good idea that I may have a lower count, so I was mentally prepared for some issues – but this? It was a real shock.

From the outset it was clear that the GPs were out of their depth giving news on such an emotive subject. After I eventually plucked up the courage and went for some tests, I was told the results by a doctor with very poor English and an even worse bedside manner. 'They're all dead,' he said, referring to my sperm. We asked to see a different doctor and he brought up the test results on the screen. I saw a word there – 'azoospermia' – and I thought: 'I've seen that before and it's not good.' He confirmed that they'd found literally no sperm at all and that I should go for another test, but shouldn't really expect to be fathering any children. And then he packed me off on my way.

We were effectively left alone to deal with this most severe blow without any support at all and it was then that I turned to the Internet for help. We found solace posting on the Fertility Friends website.

Kate and I talked endlessly about what we would and would not be prepared to do but until you are actually faced with the decision you can never say never. My first thoughts were that if it transpired that I was infertile due to genetic issues, we would not pursue the whole invasive testicle surgery, as I did not think that we would be able to cope with the stress of the low percentage chance of success, the long waits and the financial burden. I seemed to have a dodgy set of genes anyway, and from what I had read, there was the possibility of further genetic defects being passed on. I was more comfortable with donated sperm just from this genetic perspective alone. I expected that it would be a bitter pill to swallow to think that I may not be able to look into the eyes of a child that I had fathered myself, but any child is a gift, and it would be loved infinitely regardless of who provided what would have been my half of the genes.

We had been alone with our thoughts and fears for what seemed like an eternity when we were finally referred to Care Fertility in Nottingham and had the opportunity for some much-needed counselling. I was concerned that it would be like emptying a bucket of water, the emotions coming spilling out. I found that thought slightly frightening. Perhaps it is a man thing.

After a lot of soul searching I concluded that any child, born of my genes or not, would be a stranger in the sense that it may not look like me, it may not like what I like, it may grow to be 6ft 6in or 5ft 1in. The point is that my whole future has always been imaginary and, in truth, I have not lost anything other than how my children will come into this world.

I did have some concerns about the donor – I wanted the man who would be providing what would have been my half of the genetic material to be someone I felt a connection with. I got quite angry after I filled in the form that just asked me about my eye and hair colour and build, etc. I felt I was much more than just those simple physical details. Further down the line, once you have a basic match, you do get told much more about the potential donor such as occupation, hobbies, etc, which made me feel a little bit better. I've since found out that the donor sometimes writes a goodwill message to the donor-conceived child and the parents that can fill in some of the mystery, but this is only available once the child is born.

It did take me a while to come to terms with using donor sperm – you have to grieve for your lost fertility, grieve for the child that's lost in your mind. We went through some tough times. Kate was very, very upset, which I found extremely difficult, as it was effectively me or, more to the point, my body, that was causing her pain. I felt it was my role to make sure she was okay. Up until we saw the counsellor, I didn't focus on anything other than work and the little practical milestones in the process. I don't actually think I fully dealt with it emotionally until Thomas was born.

For any men wondering how they will feel about the birth of their baby created using a donor, I can honestly say that it did not cross my mind once. I was just so happy that both mother and baby were okay. I see so much of my wife in his little face. He is my little boy and that is that. I talk to him all the time and I feel so close to him already.

My child came into this world due to the actions of a very kind man and a woman who means more to me than I ever knew possible. When my child was born, I saw the face of the person I love most in the whole wide world reflected back at me. From that point onward, we began the journey to get to know each other.

Having Thomas has been so amazing; I feel that I owe something back. I do some work with the DCN, and I've signed up to be a facilitator for some of their groups. Kate is going to be an egg donor and we're planning to do egg-share IVF using the same donor sperm to have a full sibling for Thomas. When he was younger, I thought I definitely didn't want another, as I couldn't imagine loving another being as much as Thomas. However, now I would like another child, not only to complete my family but also for Thomas to have someone else to share the journey with.

If I were to give any advice, it would be, speak to someone as soon as possible about how you are feeling. Demand that the doctor sort out some counselling as you will really need to deal with the emotional fallout. Men generally find it very difficult to talk, but try not to clam up. Keep talking to your partner as you will have to make some tough choices together. The other piece of advice is, try not to think ahead too far. Bite-sized chunks are much easier to deal with. Cope with what you need to for the immediate future. Once your child is in your arms, you will realise just how special they are, how amazing your partner is and how much they mean to you.

Pip Reilly describes the experience of counselling infertile men as analogous to working on a jigsaw puzzle. He explains: 'You start by examining what's there, all the feelings and fears, then you try to put the jigsaw back together so there's clarity. And with the clarity, you can put back some coping strategies. That's the end of the process.'

What coping strategies does he normally work with?
The typical thing I ask is, 'What do you love doing? What did you last laugh about? When did you last really relax – what were you doing?' So you work out what they love and from that you can devise a coping strategy that will take them onto the next level. Whatever works: it's their journey.

CHAPTER 8

CHANGING PERSPECTIVES: EMBRACING REALITY

"The art of living lies less in eliminating our troubles than in growing with them."
Bernard M Baruch

―――――――――――――

For much of the twentieth century, the universal self-help slogan was 'Think positive'. Therapists and coaches, many from the USA, inspired conference halls full of people with the idea that they could achieve whatever they wanted, so long as they had the right attitude. If you could dream it, you could do it.

But the problem arose when people attributed more power to positive thoughts than was justifiable. If your dream failed to come true, it was because your attitude was faulty. Now coaches are challenging that premise, as it can cause people who are already suffering from events beyond their control to feel even more victimised. You aren't pregnant yet? Well, you obviously haven't been thinking happy enough thoughts. That may sound a bit facetious, but there is a lot of literature out there that claims the impossible, and people in a vulnerable state, such as those going through multiple IVF cycles, are an easy target for would-be 'miracle baby-makers'. This type of thinking can be extremely damaging for someone who may not end up with the biological child they are longing for. How much better it would be to channel the power of positive thoughts into living a full and happy life, whatever comes your way.

Of course, I'm making it sound easy. None of it is. Even the most optimistic people have bad days. They could have a sunny disposition by nature, or they could have worked hard on themselves. Either way, what all the most vivacious people I know share is the ability to be realistic, and to feel all their emotions, both positive and negative. And those embarking on fertility treatment will be experiencing more highs and lows than the average individual.

In this chapter, we'll be looking at what happens when things don't go according to plan. If you are coming to the point where you have decided 'enough is enough' – or your body/partner's body has made that decision for you – I hope that the inspirational women you will meet in the following pages will offer some comfort. You may be asking yourself, 'How do I know when I've reached the end of the line?' Nobody can answer that question but you and your partner. You may want to revisit that decision later on. But if, for now, you are willing to contemplate what a future without biological children might look and feel like, read on.

A recent Dutch study looked for the first time at the psychological effect that IVF treatment has on women in the long term. Those who were unsuccessful tended to adapt in one of four ways: continuing to pursue medical options to have a biological child; still having a desire for a child but not pursuing it actively; pursuing alternative ways of having a child (for example, adoption); or focusing on new life goals. The researchers found that 'significantly higher levels of anxiety and depression were found in the two groups still pursuing a desire for pregnancy … compared with the two groups of women who had abandoned their active pursuit of pregnancy' (those focusing on new life goals and alternative ways of having a family such as adoption).

Interestingly, it also found that 'in general, couples seem to adjust to their infertility', a process that the researchers estimate takes about two years – the same amount of time experts say it takes to grieve a death.

The women's levels of depression and anxiety actually returned to the baseline recorded at the start of treatment, indicating that unsuccessful IVF does not necessarily cause long-term psychological harm, but that continued attempts to become pregnant increased negative feelings.

It concludes that 'helping women to change life goals after abandoning treatment might have beneficial effects on the adaptation process', and recommends that 'clinicians could address the issue of abandoning treatment in their final consultations and inform patients about the emotional consequences of letting go of their attempts to get pregnant. Indicating that grief is a natural response might help patients to understand their emotions. In addition, the prospect of most women adjusting well after several years might encourage them to give up treatment and focus on other life goals'.

This might not be what you want to hear. I wish I could wave a magic wand and help you create what you most desire. But at the beginning of this book, I promised that I could help you make the most of your life, whether your treatment was successful or not. I believe that life is for living and we can't know what the future holds. We can only confront each challenge with the knowledge that we are doing the best we can at each moment - and be gentle with ourselves in feeling all the emotions that come our way. There is a wonderful book by Susan Jeffers called *Embracing Uncertainty*,[2] which includes some excellent exercises on making the most of life when you have no idea what the future holds - which, of course, none of us, even those with children, do.

The two people you are about to meet have made very different journeys to the place they are currently at, both living lives without the children they desperately wanted. They are strong, inspirational women whose stories reflect the pain of confronting a life that differed greatly from their dreams.

CASE STUDY

Lesley is an actor and drama teacher who spent most of her thirties receiving treatment for infertility caused by a drug her mother had taken while pregnant to prevent her miscarrying. DES (diethylstilbestrol) was given to many women in the UK from the 1950s to the 1970s, but was subsequently found to render many of their daughters infertile and at greater risk of certain types of cancer, abnormalities of the cervix, uterus and fallopian tubes, and a number of autoimmune diseases. In the USA, millions have been affected by DES and a large percentage of men and women have struggled with infertility as a result.

LESLEY'S STORY

I wouldn't say I have come to terms with it, and I don't think I ever will. You negotiate with it all the time and you might have a set of rules that you don't speak aloud, but you work out how and where to deal with it every day. Maybe that's my version of 'coming to terms'.

I started treatment at the age of 32, when Louise Brown, the first IVF baby, was five years old, and finished at 40. I had promised myself that I would stop then for the sake of any baby's health, and because I knew that if I did not put a boundary in place, I would not be able to take a positive decision and might go on trying to find the money for treatment. I think my husband would have taken the decision earlier because he saw what it was doing to me.

By the time we realised that our chances of conceiving, even with medical intervention, were low, we were too old to adopt a very young child in England. For many reasons, we decided that we were not the right people to adopt an older child. I felt guilty about this because there are so many children in care who could do with a 'family' home. We thought about inter-country adoption but were unsure about taking children out of their own culture. I felt that my need to have a child shouldn't be at the expense of them having to cope later with all the difficulties of dislocation, although that was some years ago and I think people probably have a better understanding now of the issues raised in that situation. We confessed to each other a couple of years ago that the thing we hadn't explored properly was fostering. It has greater difficulties in some ways than adoption, but we felt it was more of a 'job' and that as teachers we might have understood more easily how to work in this way with older children.

During my forties, I was very split as a personality. I have always been extremely active and sociable, so people who didn't know me well probably wouldn't have known how depressed I was. I would work 12–14 hours a day, and at one point I felt I was running four or five lives at the same time. But I don't think I was really coping. I put myself into analytic therapy just before the end of treatment and although it was helpful, I don't think I ever really talked about being childless and what it meant. My therapist was careful because I was in a bad state and I probably wasn't ready to talk about it – but I would have talked to women who had been through it, the ones who were in my situation. I had phoned the hospital before and they had put me in touch with someone who had been through treatment without success – but she actually had a biological child already so that was no help to me.

There are very few people in this country who have been affected by DES, in comparison with the USA, where there are millions – so I belong to a support group based over there. I also joined More to Life, which is part of Infertility Network UK. I had resisted being a member for a long time but when I started shouting at dinner parties I realised that I needed to talk to other childless women. People share so much on the forum. One of the things I think we need to talk about, even while going through treatment, is when and how to end it; about what happens if it 'fails'.

The issue of post-traumatic stress disorder needs to be looked into in relation to fertility treatment, with its constant building up and letting down of expectations, again and again. I wonder if people who are prone to depression, like myself, are especially in need of regular support during treatment. The mourning process is not all elegant black garments; it is often messy, violently red with anger and full of the bile of envy, before you get to the sadness. There is great comfort in going through this in the company of people who know the situation from the inside. I would constantly compare myself with other women, particularly mothers, and find myself wanting. I still do. I try to keep my achievements in mind all the time and remember I have done things.

For some people, the idea of joining a support group might not be appropriate at this stage, but it can be reassuring to know that there are other women out there in a similar situation. They deliver words of comfort that only someone else who's 'been there' can.

CASE STUDY

Rachel understands the power of sharing and listening – she spoke to more than sixty women about their experiences while researching her book on childlessness. But twenty years ago, as a successful businesswoman with a new husband she adored, it never occurred to her that she would never have the family she dreamt of. A year after their wedding, her husband dropped the bombshell that he didn't – nor ever would – want children. Devastated, Rachel spent the next four months trying to make a decision. Should she stay or should she go?

RACHEL'S STORY

It was the hardest decision I've ever had to make. I lived on a knife edge. I would try out the two different scenarios and 'live' with the feelings for a few days so I could see what staying or leaving would feel like. In the end, I decided to stay because I loved him and we worked well together. I thought that was the end – we'd have the most un-child-friendly house you could possibly imagine, we'd buy a sports car, have exotic holidays, I'd keep my figure and we'd live the good life. But what I hadn't prepared for was how hard it would be to live emotionally with that rational decision.

I spent four years in grief, then I got to the stage where I grew tired and bored of feeling so terrible. It was like a rucksack of sorrow that I carried around and just couldn't put down. Eventually, in sheer desperation, I had some therapy and it was during one session that I realised I needed to mourn the children I would never have. Coming to see my childlessness as a bereavement was helpful. Society doesn't acknowledge the death of something that never was, but when I started reading books on bereavement that talked about emotions like anger, guilt, frustration and jealousy, I saw I was on the path of mourning that marked the beginning of my recovery.

I asked three things of my husband, which he agreed to: that I could bring up the subject of our childlessness day or night, whenever I felt the need; that we would reject any possessions that had family connotations (such as a 4x4 car); and that if anyone asked if we had children, I could reply: 'Sadly, we don't; my husband doesn't want any.'

I found sex really confusing. Living with involuntary childlessness can wreck your sex life and your libido. You can end up feeling not much of a woman if you wanted children and don't have them. My husband was quite sexually voracious and I would think: 'You're very keen on it, but not on the reason you have it.' I remember in the early days, people would ask, 'Do I hear the patter of tiny feet?' and he would say, 'No, we're just practising.' I wanted to scream out the real reason, but at the same time, I understood it was important to him that he looked virile. Of course, impotence and infertility have no connection, but to the outside world, particularly to men, they can appear to.

(Some years later, Rachel met a woman called Louise on the Greek island of Skyros, where they were both attending a personal-development workshop. In Louise, she found the perfect collaborator for a book she had imagined writing several years before but had not felt emotionally ready for. Thanks to her years as a market researcher, Rachel was able to conduct in-depth interviews with women who wanted children but who were childless, all for different reasons.)

I listened to the emotional stories of their childlessness. Many had talked their medical stories to death, but never before had they spoken in depth to another childless woman about the huge emotional cost of their situation. Listening to their struggles was a privilege; it was also hugely bonding. It's incredibly powerful, enabling women to talk about something that's rarely discussed, even with partners.

(The resulting book, Beyond Childlessness[3], *also includes interviews with counsellors who felt it was important to manage expectations early on, so people undergoing IVF view ending up with a baby as just one of the possible outcomes, while not having children is another.)*

When I went to interview a counsellor at one fertility clinic, there was a large, laminated piece of pink paper on the noticeboard in the waiting room, put up by a client. It said, 'We had six failed IVF treatments and the seventh succeeded', and she now has the most adorable twins or triplets – the message being, never give up. I nearly tore it down, I was so angry. I thought: 'How dare you? How dare you give these men and women coming here false hope?'

I also interviewed women with unexplained infertility, and they would say that the most difficult decision was when to call it a day. When they and their partner had finally come to that place, the consultant would often say: 'Well, that's your decision, but if you change your mind you can always come back and have another go.' So they received no support for what, for many, was the hardest decision of their lives.

The trouble is that these women's lives are on ice; they're just existing, waiting to get pregnant. That's the real awfulness of it. It can ruin your relationships with your partner, your family, your friends, and it can ruin your health. A very important thing, especially in the beginning, is to work out what you want to say when people ask if you have children. You might want to rehearse your reply. There is no single right response, just what feels right for you at the time. But then you may want to review it, at first every six months, then maybe every year or two, as you work through a phase. So you might start by simply saying, 'No, I don't', and, later, you might want to say, 'Sadly, we couldn't, my tubes are blocked', or whatever is appropriate to your situation.

If you have children, you have a ready-made purpose and role in life. And if you wanted them and don't have any, you may feel an incredible void that, at the beginning, you can never imagine being filled. There is no instant path to follow: you have to search for a purpose, and you can find it in many different ways. I spoke to one woman for my book, a journalist who goes to war zones, who believes she has a privilege that a parent does not – that if she dies on the job, her death, while sad for friends and family, would not be 'irresponsible'. I know someone else who mentors a child in a children's home, giving her fun days out and helping her face challenges. It's about ploughing your own furrow, whether it's tending your garden or cycling round the world. You have to find what's right for you.

(When I was talking to Rachel, she was about to leave for a remote part of northern Namibia, where she teaches public speaking to primary-school children and their teachers. She is also a godmother – something she was never able to contemplate during the early years – is recently divorced, and now has a new partner with teenage children. She is entering another phase – grandchildlessness.)

The very last thing I said in my book is that I saw myself as a proud survivor of my childlessness, and when I wrote that, it felt brilliant, like I had planted a flag on top of Everest. Then, about 18 months after I had said that and felt so proud, the next step of the journey revealed itself, and I thought: 'If I keep saying to myself, "I'm a non-mother and that's okay," I'm putting my childlessness at the centre of my identity.' So I said to myself: 'Okay, you've done that now – what are you going to be if not a mother?' That's my new journey. It's exciting and it's still revealing itself to me. I've come to realise there are so many more ways to nurture and to live a joyful, fulfilling life apart from motherhood.

Exercise: finding your purpose

Purpose is a loaded word – and for good reason. It implies that you, as an individual, have a meaning in this world, something you can achieve through a combination of your actions and your personality. Some people have always had a clear sense of purpose, and see it as a calling or vocation. Others might never have thought about it before. Either way, only you can decide what it is. The following exercise, which is from the life coach Fiona Harrold's book *The 7 Rules of Success*, provides an excellent starting point in identifying your vision. Where you take it beyond that is up to you.

Answer these simple questions with a short statement for each:

1. What do you want most out of life? Try to think of this as a state of being, rather than a specific thing, such as a baby (for example, to be happy and fulfilled).

2. What do you want to see happen in the world (for example, peace and happiness)?
3. What makes you special (for example, my energy, drive and enthusiasm, ability to inspire and motivate others)?
4. What things can you do/are you capable of doing right now (for example, writing, public speaking, coaching)?

Now write this statement as follows:
I will ... (choose one answer from 4), using my ... (answer from 3), to accomplish ... (answer from 2), and in doing so achieve ... (answer from 1).
For example: *I will write and speak using my ability to inspire and motivate to accomplish peace and happiness and in so doing achieve joy and fulfilment.*

Adoption

For some people, the 'A word' is seriously taboo when they're experiencing fertility issues, though I imagine many will have at least contemplated it. It's perfectly understandable that, given all the time, physical and emotional energy, and often money you have spent trying to become pregnant, you may view adoption as 'inferior' to having a biological child. However, if you're at the stage where you think you could be coming to the end of the line in terms of treatment, but still know that you want to be a parent, it's worth giving it proper consideration.

Most agencies ask couples who have been undergoing fertility treatment to wait at least a year before starting the adoption process, to give them time to grieve fully and think things over. But there is no harm in gathering information and having a look at websites such as BAAF's (British Association for Adoption & Fostering)[4] for facts and personal stories from people who have trodden the path before you.

BAAF's Esther Freeman says: 'Infertility is one of the most common reasons people come to adoption and many of them have had a difficult journey.' But what can start as a 'last resort' for couples who have experienced the agony of unsuccessful treatment can soon turn into something unexpectedly wonderful. As Esther says: 'People fall in love every day with other people who aren't biologically related to them. Although some say that blood is thicker than water, you'll hear many adoptive parents say that love is thicker than blood.'

CASE STUDY

Here is the story of Carole's journey. For her, adoption marked the closing of one door and the opening of another onto a life happier than she could ever have imagined.

CAROLE'S STORY

We started trying to get pregnant in October 1997, a year after we were married. It wasn't happening, so I threw myself into holistic therapies, as I really wanted to conceive naturally. I tried everything – reflexology, massage, hypnotherapy, healing, the Bowen technique [which stimulates the body to rebalance itself], anything I thought might help.

I was determined not to do IVF. Before we were married, Andy and I watched a TV programme about it and I said to him: 'If we can't have children, we'll just have to accept it, as I'll never put myself through that.' But of course it's different when you get there. Eventually, as it just wasn't happening, we decided to do an IVF cycle as a way of seeing if anything was wrong. It turned out that not only was everything fine, but I had the egg levels of someone in her twenties (I was in my early thirties at this point) and my husband had a high sperm count. We were highly fertile and the consultants said it should be a textbook procedure: there was no reason why it shouldn't work.

We were offered counselling at the clinic but didn't feel we needed it. I had good support from the Babyworld.co.uk forum, where I'd been a member for several years. We all shared our emotions online, whether we were going through a good or a bad time, and that was a godsend for me – you're talking to these people every day. Family and friends don't understand as they've never been through it, and here you have 20-plus women to talk to who are in the same situation as you.

When the IVF failed, Andy and I stuck together like glue – other people didn't get a look in. We were in such pain, and platitudes from well-meaning friends didn't help. I'd go to the shopping centre, see a pregnant woman and burst into tears, and have to come home again. That's why we kept ourselves to ourselves in the first few months after treatment – we just couldn't face people and deal with what they had to say.

There were two embryos remaining and we couldn't leave them, so a year later we did a frozen embryo transfer (FET), but I had a feeling it wouldn't work – and it didn't.

It didn't take as long to get over as the IVF, partly because I wasn't as full of hormones from the egg stimulation. I respond badly to hormones (ironically, I was never able to take the pill), which is why we decided to do only one IVF cycle. We were both certain about that. What was harder was letting go of trying naturally for a baby, especially as there was nothing wrong and it could, theoretically, happen at any time. I can't pinpoint exactly when we said, 'Enough's enough', but we were sure at the time we weren't going to adopt. We just decided we would be a couple that goes on holiday and has lovely cars.

It wasn't that easy, though – I would still brace myself for that phone call from friends telling me they were pregnant. A friend from college had three children in the time I was trying. You do lose friendships along the way, as your lives are so different. I was lucky, though, as my closest friends either didn't want children or had older ones, so I wasn't surrounded by babies and bumps the whole time. It was hard when it came to my family – my brother had a little boy, but my way of dealing with it was to throw myself into looking after him. I didn't think it would help but it did, and it gave me my 'baby fix'. He's still the apple of my eye.

A couple of years after the FET, I bumped into someone at work who was leaving at the end of the week because she was adopting two children. I'd read so many horror stories about adoption, I was really interested in her experience. She said it was 'nowhere near as bad as an IVF cycle' and that stuck in my mind. It seemed there were a lot of myths about – for example, that you can't adopt a baby when you're over 35. It's more to do with the availability of younger children and the number of adopters wanting infants. I went home and asked my husband what he thought. He said we should wait until the following year, but we decided to do some research and send off for an information pack.

We were determined not to rush things. I set up an adoption forum on Babyworld so I could talk to people who were going through the process. Before the prep course even started, I almost pulled out. I thought: 'Are we playing with fire here? We're a happy couple – shouldn't we just accept our fate?'

Social workers give you the worst-case scenarios, and it's quite scary before you get into the process and understand it. I wasn't sure if we could take on a child with special needs; most adopted children do have special needs and they all need patience in varying degrees.

We did end up going on the prep course but I was still fixated on conceiving. Of course, everyone says: 'Now you're adopting, you'll get pregnant.' But you are told quite firmly that you have to use contraception as you can't become pregnant when you're actually in the process of adopting a child. They like to know you've come to terms with your infertility and you won't be pursuing further treatment. But they don't expect you never to have a twinge if you see a pregnant woman or never to have regrets about not having a biological child. They want you to be human and to have had life experiences so you can empathise with a child who may have been through difficult times.

Our light-bulb moment was when we went to the panel and were faced with 12 people asking us questions about our ability to parent an adopted child. I likened that panel day to getting a positive pregnancy test – not that I'd know how that feels. That was the moment I thought: 'At last, we're going to be parents.' And a few months later our new baby came home with us, a nine-month old girl.

I would urge anyone considering adoption to research it fully and not to rely on what you read in magazines or see on TV. You could be missing out on a good thing by thinking you already know what it's all about.

It's difficult to tell someone when it's time to move on from fertility treatment. I think you just know. You have to make a choice between living your life with regrets and sadness, being happy with what you have, or making the baby thing happen in another way.

I would never do IVF again but I don't regret it, because it brought us to where we are today. When I see people having treatment, I think: 'If only you knew how brilliant adoption is.' But they have to go through the process themselves. Not everyone has a success story, but I do know a lot of adopters and not one of them would change a thing.

AFTERWORD

Congratulations on having come this far. I hope that, by now, you are feeling less alone, more aware of your inner resources and confident in your ability to invest in your life, whatever your situation. I also hope you will be feeling compassionate towards yourself and your partner, and stronger in your sense of self and as a couple. My biggest thrill when I see clients is that light-bulb moment when they realise they have more inside them than they ever thought. They often arrive feeling, 'I can't do it, it's all too difficult', and by the end they're well into an IVF cycle, doing things they never thought they could and celebrating the little victories they rightly own.

I would love to end this book on a neat and tidy note, but I can't. For a start, I sincerely hope it doesn't feel like an ending – more like the beginning of an exciting new chapter of your life. And regardless of your circumstances – whether you have decided to start treatment, stop treatment, look at other options or are even pregnant already – it is natural to feel doubt and, perhaps, a little fear. This is the nature of change, as we mourn the loss of what can often come to seem familiar and even comforting. I have known women feel ambivalent when they finally become pregnant after many years of struggle. They had been someone who was 'trying for a baby', and took on all the feelings and attitudes they associated with that situation. Once they no longer had that identity, assuming a new one, of 'mother-to-be', felt strange and uncomfortable.

Luckily, we are always changing, and even when things seem to be stuck, we are actually preparing ourselves for something new, however unconscious the process. Knowing this can help you to stay in the present moment and become truly aware of the power you have to shape your future. I hope that the exercises in this book and the stories you have heard have inspired you to embrace the change and feel a greater sense of control in your life as you continue on your journey.

If I could leave you with just three thoughts, I would urge you to remember the following:

■ Please, please don't underestimate the seriousness of infertility. It is a real emotional and physical shock to the system and your feelings need to be acknowledged. Don't think you 'should' be coping better, and don't let anyone else tell you as much. It is a major trauma and you must understand that. Only then is it really possible to start being kind to yourself and look at coping strategies.

■ Just because you've reached the end of this book doesn't mean you should put it in a drawer and never look at it again. Keep using the tools and exercises – they work, whatever your life situation. I spoke recently to a client I hadn't seen in years, and she was still using some of the techniques, even though our sessions had finished and her fertility treatment was successful. I often use them myself, to keep me focused and in touch with my feelings. Life can get so busy that it's easy to lose track of who we are and what we want. These tools and exercises will help refocus the mind and refresh the spirit.

■ The fact is that most people who want to will manage to create a family somehow or other, even if it's not as straightforward as they'd initially hoped. When I was going through my years of infertility, I stuck a Post-it note above my mirror to reassure me in the difficult moments. It read: 'Everything will be okay in the end. And if it's not okay, it's not the end.'

I wish you all the best with your journey – may you find that place where it's all okay in the end.

REFERENCES

Chapter 1
1. Encyclopedia of Alternative Medicine, 2005: Journal Therapy
2. 999 Reasons to Laugh at Infertility (www.999reasonstolaugh.com)
3. Winston, R. *A Child Against All Odds*, Bantam Press, 2006, p 150

Chapter 2
1. Ryan, C. 'Hypnosis 'doubles IVF success'', *BBC News Online*, 2004
2. Sample, I. 'Cutting stress may increase chances of pregnancy', *The Guardian*, 21st June, 2006
3. www.domarcenter.com

Chapter 4
1. Casiday, R. et al. *Volunteering and Health: What impact does it really have?* University of Lampeter and Volunteering England, 2008

Chapter 6
1. Love, P. and Stosny, S. *Why Women Talk and Men Walk*, Vermilion, 2007

Chapter 7
1. Lee, S. *Counselling in Male Infertility*, Blackwell, 1996
2. www.mensfe.net
3. www.donor-conception-network.org

Chapter 8
1. Verhaak, C.M. et al. 'Long-term psychological adjustment to IVF / ICSI treatment', *Human Reproduction*, vol 22, no. 1, 2007, pp. 305–308

2. Jeffers, S. *Embracing Uncertainty*, Hodder Mobius, 2003
3. Black, R. and Scull, L. *Beyond Childlessness*, Rodale International, 2005
4. www.baaf.org.uk

FURTHER RESOURCES

General infertility support and information

The Infertility Network UK **www.infertilitynetwork.com** (advice and information about infertility)

BICA **www.bica.net** (counselling for infertility)

Fertility Friends **www.fertilityfriends.co.uk** (help and support for those undergoing treatment)

HFEA **www.hfea.gov.uk** (regulatory authority for fertility treatment)

BACP **www.bacp.co.uk** (association for counselling and therapy, offers a search function for accredited counsellors)

Specialist conditions

Miscarriage Association **www.miscarriageassociation.org.uk** (support and advice about miscarriage)

The Daisy Network **www.daisynetwork.org.uk** (premature menopause)

SANDS **www.uk-sands.org** (Stillbirth and neonatal death support)

Verity **www.verity-pcos.org.uk** (Information and support about PCOS)

Ashermans **www.ashermans.org** (Miscarriage through intrauterine adhesions)

Donor Conception Network **www.donor-conception-network.org**

Men

Mensfe.net **www.mensfe.net** (support for infertile men)

Alternative therapies

The Kite Clinic **www.kiteclinic.co.uk**

Foresight **www.foresight-preconception.org.uk**

British Acupuncture Council **www.acupuncture.org.uk**

Adoption and fostering

British Association for Adoption and Fostering **www.baaf.org.uk**; **www.bemyparent.org.uk**

Other support

More to Life **www.infertilitynetworkuk.com/moretolife/**

Beyond Childlessness **www.beyondchildlessness.com**

Personal development

Powerchange Personal Development Service
www.powerchange.com

Fiona Harrold Life coaching **www.fionaharrold.com**

Miscellaneous

Volunteer Centres **www.volunteering.org.uk www.do-it.org**

INDEX

17629792R00071

Made in the USA
San Bernardino, CA
14 December 2014